# GERRY'S
# REAL WORLD GUIDE
# TO
# PHARMACOKINETICS
# & OTHER THINGS

# GERRY'S REAL WORLD GUIDE TO PHARMACOKINETICS & OTHER THINGS

By

G. M. Woerlee MBBS (W. Aust), FRCA (Lond.)

*Anesthesiologist*

*Rijnland Hospital, Leiderdorp, the Netherlands*

Disclaimer:
This is a textbook presented in the form of a work of fiction. Accordingly, the locations, characters and events in this book are fictitious. Any similarities to actual locations, or real persons, either living or dead, are coincidental and not intended by the author. As regards the medical data and calculations, every effort has been made to ensure the accuracy of the information presented in this book. Furthermore, any person using data contained in this book should realize that medical data is always subject to inter-individual variation, as well as ensuring they have checked their own calculations before proceeding with any medical treatments. The publishers accept no responsibility for any inaccuracies contained within this text.

Printed in the United States of America.

Booklocker.com, Inc.
2008

# Contents

# Preface

Anesthesiologists are regularly bombarded with pharmacokinetic and pharmacodynamic data about the drugs they use. Some pay attention to these data, using these data to guide them in their choice and use of drugs. Yet others ignore these data, simply asking their colleagues and pharmaceutical company representatives, "How can I best use this drug? How much should I administer? How long will it work?" Both approaches have their merits. In fact, when asked, both groups will actually use anesthetic drugs in a similar manner. So why bother learning anything about the pharmacokinetic and pharmacodynamic properties of drugs, when an empirical approach works just as well? By now the reader will have noticed I used the word pharmacokinetic three times, just as I also used the word pharmacodynamic three times in this paragraph. But what do these terms mean?

- Pharmacokinetics is the mathematical and qualitative description of the distribution of drugs within the body, as well as their elimination from the body.
- Pharmacodynamics is the mathematical and qualitative description of the effects of drugs upon the organ systems of the body.

There are good reasons for understanding and using the pharmacokinetic and pharmacodynamic properties of drugs. One of the most important reasons is that a purely empirical approach means that learning how to use any drug safely and appropriately entails a long and inefficient period of trial and error. Indeed, while writing this preface, I was reminded of a piece of advice in an old book on practical anesthesia, in which the authors advised that because suprapubic prostatectomy is not especially painful, all that was required for adequate anesthesia was intravenous Thiopental, sometimes supplemented with Meperidine. Most modern anesthesiologists would fall over backwards with astonishment upon reading this. But at the time this advice was given, the usual anesthetic intravenous induction doses of Thiopental were very high—high enough to induce coma in nearly all people, with the resulting unresponsiveness to pain, which is why few patients ever reacted to the pain of the operation. Such doses of Thiopental were also high enough to induce severe myocardial depression, vasodilatation, and even lethal shock in some patients. Such salutary near-lethal, and actual lethal experiences, eventually taught anesthesiologists to use lower Thiopental doses, upon which they discovered that suprapubic prostatectomy really was painful. This is an example of empirical determination of drug use.

Understanding of pharmacokinetics and pharmacodynamics offers a better way. Known and unfamiliar drugs can be used more efficiently and safely, and their clinical effects are readily understood. Moreover, understanding of the pharmacokinetic and pharmacodynamic properties of current anesthetic drugs makes it possible to devise new ways of using these drugs. Knowledge of the pharmacokinetic and pharmacodynamic properties of new drugs makes it possible to calculate whether they offer more advantages than existing drugs, as well as their initial applications and dosage regimes—all of which considerably reduces the amount of trial and error needed to learn to use such new drugs, or whether it is worthwhile using them at all.

This book is written for all those wishing to learn about just these basic principles of pharmacokinetics and pharmacokinetics as applied to anesthetic drugs. It is intended as a light, easily read, and hopefully entertaining guide teaching these things with a maximum of practical common sense and a minimum of mathematical knowledge. It does not pretend to offer the nirvana of total knowledge and control. Such knowledge and such control are dreams. But what the interested reader will find is a path, a way of thinking and doing—a Real World Guide to Pharmacokinetics & Other Things. These "Other Things" are intended to give readers some insights into the ways basic physiology, pharmacokinetics, and pharmacodynamics can be applied to the questions and wondrous phenomena confronting them each day during their clinical duties. In other words, this is a book written for anesthesiologists, consultant or specialist anesthesiologists, residents, senior registrars, registrars, senior house officers, and anesthetic nurses. For the sake of simplicity I will call the average reader a resident, the American term for a doctor undergoing postgraduate specialization.

Some people may say that the pharmacokinetic and pharmacodynamic concepts in this book could all be summarized on four pages. I fully agree, but years of experience have taught me that very few residents ever really learn these concepts in this way. My personal experience is that concepts are only truly learned, understood, and anchored in the minds of residents when accompanied by memorable practical examples illustrating those concepts. This is what I have attempted to do for each concept.

Purists may object to the use of the two-compartment pharmacokinetic model throughout this book. They will almost certainly say that, "The kinetics of many anesthetic drugs are more accurately described by a three-compartment model." They are quite correct—but only to a certain degree. A two-compartment pharmacokinetic model makes it possible to perform simple, but clinically relevant calculations in situations of intermittent intravenous bolus drug administration and short intravenous infusions—methods of drug use in more than 95% of all general anesthetics administered throughout the world. Furthermore, this model is an invaluable aid enabling students to understand the practical applications of pharmacokinetic and pharmacodynamic principles, so making it a useful way to learn and apply these concepts to clinical practice—the fundamental purpose of this book. Those who understand these principles, possess computers and have a desire to perform more complex calculations, can always progress to pharmacokinetic models with more compartments and complexity.

Some people may object to the irreverent, even flippant way I have illustrated situations in the operating theater. To these people I can only say that such is the daily reality of all those who work in operating theaters. People working in operating theaters are regularly confronted with the sights, sounds, and stench of human disease and degradation. Personal mental survival in such situations is only possible with humor and perspective, together with the will to perform good work. Those who wish to view these things in a more religious and philosophical perspective may always do so, but they too are confronted with, and must somehow mentally cope with the same problems. A recent book of mine called "Mortal Minds" is a way of coping with the problems presented by human degradation, disease, and mortality by providing a definitive physiological basis for humanistic philosophy.

I enjoyed writing this book, because it is an expression of the world I experience each working day. True, there is a slightly Dutch flavor to some of the situations, but having personally worked in Australia, England, as well as in The Netherlands, I know language, accents, and geography may differ, but the situations sketched are similar in all modern Western hospitals. I am sure many of my intended readers will recognize, and hopefully be amused by these same situations and experiences.

I gratefully acknowledge the assistance of Dr. F. Engbers, Dr. K. Burger, Dr. F. Wilkinson, Dr. I. Dons, and Dr. T. Vd Ende for providing invaluable encouragement and feedback on initial versions of the manuscript. The group practice in which I practice anesthesia, as well as my clinical work in the Rijnland Hospital in Leiderdorp, have been a continual source of questions and problems that could only adequately be answered by the approach taken in this book. Finally, and most importantly, I wish to thank my wife, Johanna Woerlee-van Horn, for her patience and understanding while this short monograph came into being.

G. M. Woerlee
Leiden, The Netherlands,
October 2008

# 1

# Bob

A bustle of blue clad people heralded the beginning of a new day in the operating theaters of Saint Elders Hospital. Scrub nurses walked around pushing trolleys loaded high with packages of instruments and drapes. Anesthesiologists and their assistants checked their instruments, machines, drugs, and infusions before rushing off to drink a cup of coffee prior to beginning with their operating lists. The first patients began arriving in the holding area. It was a normal start to a normal day.

Yet this day was different. It was the start of the new teaching year for the anesthetic residents. Doctor Bob was one of these residents, now in his third year of the anesthetic training program of Saint Elders Hospital. His mentor for this year was Doctor Gerry, an experienced crusty older anesthesiologist, known as a teacher intolerant of fools, especially of those lacking any desire to learn. He was also known to be a bit of a pharmacokinetic freak. Doctor Bob was a bit worried about this. He had followed lectures on pharmacokinetics and pharmacodynamics. He had even bought a book on these subjects. Even so, his understanding of the practical aspects of these subjects was still rather hazy. All he had actually learned from the rather uninspired lectures, and from the very complex and highly mathematical book, were that pharmacokinetics and pharmacodynamics were devilishly complex and arcane sciences with seemingly little relation to the very practical business of administering anesthesia, a specialism he enjoyed, and was even getting good at. So Bob approached this first day with some trepidation, because he knew from his colleagues that his mentor would start asking tricky questions on the first day—a bit like how a barking dog would test a stranger.

Bob met Doctor Gerry in the coffee room. Gerry was drinking strong black coffee while leafing through a popular daily newspaper. His first reaction upon seeing Bob was to grunt, "You're late. Don't like that. Begin on time, and you'll finish on time—preferably at a civilized time in the afternoon. I hate finishing in the dark. I hate going home in the dark. I want to see daylight at least once a day. Be on time tomorrow to check your machines, drugs, and instruments. I've already done it for you today. You do it from tomorrow. Now have a cup of coffee. Nothing like a caffeine jolt to start the day."

After excusing himself and explaining why he was late, Bob drank his coffee and accompanied his mentor to the operating theater. The first patient was there already, a portly middle-aged man of Mediterranean origin called Mr. Terra who was to undergo an open cholecystectomy under general anesthesia. He was extremely anxious despite premedication with a relatively high dose of Lorazepam: he perspired profusely, his pupils were wide open, and he had hypertension together with tachycardia. After a fruitless attempt at reassuring and calming the man, Gerry and Bob induced anesthesia.

Terra was certainly unconscious and under adequate general anesthesia, yet his heart rate and blood pressure remained high. Doctor George Curvoisier—a surgeon who prided himself on the speed with which he could perform an old-fashioned open cholecystectomy—began the operation. Gerry looked at the monitors, looked over the drapes into the wound to check that the operating conditions were good, that the blood was not cyanotic, and that the surgeon had everything under control. He then left without a word. Bob was somewhat disconcerted. He thought to himself, "I must have caught him on a bad day." Bob had administered anesthesia for this type of operation many times, so he proceeded to do as he normally did with such patients.

About 30 to 40 minutes after induction of anesthesia, the pulse rate and blood pressure of Mr. Terra subsided to normal levels, and shortly afterwards Courvoisier started closing the abdomen. Just then, Gerry reappeared in the operating theater, nodded to Bob, but said nothing. He looked at the wound, looked at his watch, looked at the operating list, and remarked to the surgeon, "Hey George, are you sure you don't need to re-open the patient? You've taken so long with this operation that he might have grown new stones in his bile duct again."

George replied, "If you and your residents could give even half way decent anesthesia, these operations wouldn't take anywhere near so long."

"Tsk, tsk... Pearls before swine. You really don't know how lucky you are to have me as an anesthesiologist..." George had heard all this before, sighed deeply, and continued suturing in silence. He was in no mood for further banter—he was looking forward to a cup of coffee. Gerry asked Bob to order the next patient, while at the same time asking, "Tell me Bob, what is the ideal patient turnaround time?"

Bob looked surprised, confused even. No one had ever asked him this question before, so he answered in an uncertain tone, "I don't know. I'm not quit sure what you mean."

"About 30 to 90 centimeters."

"What do you mean by 30 to 90 centimeters turnaround time?" asked a still perplexed Bob.

"I mean one patient out, and the next one coming in separated by distance of 30 to 90 centimeters. No delays that way, and we'll all be finished on time," replied Gerry as Curvoisier finished closing the skin and subsequently departed to drink coffee. Mr. Terra was aroused and extubated. Sister Hörni—a petite, quick-witted and cheerful anesthetic nurse—rang the recovery room to announce they were about to bring them a patient, only to hear that the recovery room was full. This meant Mr. Terra would have to remain in the operating theater until space was available for him in the recovery room, while the next patient would have to wait in the holding area. Mr. Terra did not seem to mind waiting—he had fallen asleep and was snoring softly. Gerry looked unhappy, sighed, and looked around with a bored expression until his eyes fell upon the anesthetic chart. Immediately his eyes lit up, and he asked, "Tell me Bob, what did you learn from this patient?"

"Uh, oh... here it comes," thought Bob, "a learning moment."

The operating theater nurses had heard similar questions in that tone from Gerry before, and hurriedly scurried off to the coffee room. They knew these learning moments always lasted at least as long as it took them to have a good gossip and a cup of coffee. Sister Hörni was unperturbed and continued with what she was doing, simply ignoring Gerry. She had heard it all before. She had already had coffee, and was now preparing anesthetic drugs and equipment for the next several patients on the operating list. She also wanted to go home on time.

"I really can't think of much," replied Bob. "It was a perfectly standard open cholecystectomy. The only unusual or different aspect to this operation was that the patient was a man, while cholecystectomy patients are usually women."

It was evident from the questioning gaze on the face of Gerry that this was not what he really wanted to hear. "And what else did you notice?" he asked.

"Er... nothing else," was the uncertain response.

"Do you ever observe and speak to the patients to whom you administer anesthesia? If you did, and if you observed this in relation to the normal physiological parameters you measure and note during each anesthetic, you would have had a wonderful lesson in applied physiology and pharmacokinetics."

Bob was silent for a few seconds before admitting, "I'm sorry, but I still don't quite know what you're trying to show me."

"I will now induct you into the wonderful world of physiological pharmacokinetics," said Gerry. "You noticed Mr. Terra was extremely anxious, possibly even terrified before we began inducing general anesthesia. His pupils were wide, he was sweating, and he had a rapid pulse as well as a high blood pressure. What are the causes of all these bodily manifestations of anxiety and fear?"

"They're all products of elevated sympathetic nervous activity together with increased secretion of epinephrine by the adrenal glands," was the rapid reply.

"And what are the effects of anesthesia on these manifestations of elevated sympathoadrenal activity?" was Gerry's equally rapid response.

Bob thought a bit before answering. "Anesthesia stops the increased sympathoadrenal activity, which means increased sympathetic nervous system activity will cease, as will increased adrenal gland secretion of epinephrine." He warmed up to his chain of logic. "However, the extra epinephrine secreted by the adrenal glands remains in the circulation, and the effects of this extra epinephrine in the circulation will continue until it is eliminated from the body."

"Very good," said Gerry. "But how long do these effects continue, and what does the duration of these effects tell us about the pharmacokinetics of epinephrine?"

Bob had a sudden inspiration. He realized that now was the time to look at Mr. Terra's anesthetic chart. He saw that Mr. Terra's blood pressure and pulse rate normalized somewhere about 30 to 40 minutes after induction of anesthesia. So he answered, "The cardiovascular effects of the increased epinephrine concentrations in the blood last about 30 to 40 minutes, which means that the half-life of epinephrine must be about 30 to 40 minutes."

"Right and wrong in that order," was Gerry's answer. "True, the effects of the extra epinephrine lasted about 30 to 40 minutes in Terra, but this does not mean the half-life of epinephrine is 30 to 40 minutes. You really must be careful about what you say about half-lives." Gerry continued, "I'll begin with the concept of a half-life. A half-life is simply the time it takes for a process to be half complete—not fully complete—but half complete. One illustration of a half-life is the well-known decay half-life of a radioactive substance, and as you implied, the concept of a half-life is also applicable to describing the pharmacokinetic properties of drugs and many other substances."

"Furthermore," continued Gerry, "when describing the pharmacokinetic properties of drugs, it is always important to remember that unless otherwise stated, concentrations of drugs in blood are always expressed as plasma drug concentrations. There are very good reasons for using plasma drug concentrations. One reason is that not all drugs can enter into erythrocytes, which means that plasma drug concentrations are not always the same as blood drug concentrations. Another reason is that drugs act on tissues outside blood vessels, and only drugs present in plasma are available for diffusion or transport into extravascular tissues. After all, drug molecules present inside erythrocytes cannot transmigrate in some miraculous way from inside erythrocytes directly into extravascular tissues—drug molecules present inside erythrocytes must first diffuse out of erythrocytes into plasma before diffusing, or being transported into extravascular tissues. This is why extravascular drug concentrations and effects are more directly related to plasma drug concentrations than to blood concentrations."

Bob interrupted, "This is all very well, but what has all this got to do with what we observed with Mr. Terra?"

"Patience young man, patience. What an impatient fellow you are. First the basics, and then all will become clear," said Gerry reprovingly. "Now we've settled a few basics, let's look at the situation of Mr. Terra. This man was anxious, very anxious prior to his operation. He wasn't anxious only in the few minutes before induction, but also anxious for some time before arriving in the operating theater. We know this from the preoperative visit, from what the ward sisters told us, and from what we saw just before induction of anesthesia. So we can make the very reasonable assumption that his adrenals secreted increased amounts of epinephrine for several hours, saturating his plasma and interstitium with above normal concentrations of epinephrine, so causing the tachycardia and hypertension we observed. Do you follow me?"

Bob nodded, "Yes. Up till now it's all quite clear, although I'm not entirely sure where you're going to. But I'm listening."

"Well here it comes. The normal plasma epinephrine concentration in calm resting adults ranges between 0.01 to 0.1 mcg/1. Epinephrine is a hormone whose effects such as tachycardia and systolic hypertension begin at plasma concentrations above the upper limit of the normal plasma epinephrine concentration range, that is above 0.1 mcg/1 in adults (1). This means that all the excess epinephrine in Mr. Terra's plasma had to be eliminated before his heart rate and blood pressure could return to normal. When the secretion of extra epinephrine into the circulation suddenly ceases, the rate of decline of the above normal plasma epinephrine concentrations is given by the plasma elimination half-life of epinephrine, which is about 11 minutes in human adults (2)."

Bob listened patiently, but upon hearing the words, plasma elimination half-life, he interrupted, "Just a minute Gerry. As you said, epinephrine doesn't cause hypertension or tachycardia by affecting plasma proteins or blood cells—epinephrine causes these effects by diffusing out of blood vessels to act on receptors on myocardial muscle cells, as well as to act on receptors on the smooth muscle cells of blood vessels. So why are we only talking about plasma concentrations? How fast does epinephrine diffuse out of blood vessels to act on extravascular tissues?"

"That's a very good question. Epinephrine is actually a small molecule that diffuses so rapidly out of capillaries that we really only need take the plasma elimination half-life into account. How do I know this? Very simply—a lot of research done many years ago showed very conclusively that human capillary endothelium forms no barrier to the diffusion of molecules whose molecular weight is less than 10,000 grams/mole (3). The molecular weight of epinephrine is 183.2 grams/mole, which means it diffuses quite rapidly through capillary endothelium. Okay there Bob?"

"Yes, it's all quite clear up till now."

"Let's return to the concept of the plasma elimination half-life. The plasma elimination half-life of a drug is a description of how fast the plasma concentration of that drug declines during the so-called elimination phase of the plasma concentration-time curve of that drug after a single bolus intravenous injection. We'll talk about wondrous things such as distribution phases and elimination phases at another time (chapter 3). Suffice to say, all you have to know and realize is that a plasma elimination half-life is not a description of how fast a drug is eliminated from the body— it is only a description of how fast that drug disappears from the plasma. Now, the plasma elimination half-life of epinephrine is about 11 minutes. Furthermore, even though Mr. Terra is under anesthesia, his adrenals still produce basal, normal amounts of epinephrine to sustain a normal plasma epinephrine concentration. So in this situation we are talking about elimination of the excess, or above normal concentrations of epinephrine in his plasma. So here is a list of what happened with Mr. Terra (also see Table 1.1)."

- After 11 minutes, the excess plasma epinephrine concentration in the blood declined by 50%, so halving the excess plasma epinephrine concentration in the blood of Mr. Terra.

- After another 11 minutes, the remaining excess plasma epinephrine concentration declined by another 50% (which is 25% of the initial excess plasma epinephrine concentration), meaning that now the excess plasma epinephrine concentration had declined by 75%, leaving the excess plasma epinephrine concentration in the blood of Mr. Terra at 25% of the initial concentration.

- After another 11 minutes, the remaining excess plasma epinephrine concentration declined by another 50% (which is 12.5% of the initial excess plasma epinephrine concentration), meaning that now the excess plasma epinephrine concentration had declined by 87.5%, leaving the excess plasma epinephrine concentration in the blood of Mr. Terra at 12.5% of the initial concentration.

- After another 11 minutes, the remaining excess plasma epinephrine concentration declined by another 50% (which is 6.25% of the initial excess plasma epinephrine concentration), meaning that now the excess plasma epinephrine concentration had declined by 93.75%, leaving the excess plasma epinephrine concentration in the blood of Mr. Terra at 6.25% of the initial concentration.

- The same method of halving continued until all the excess epinephrine was eliminated from his plasma.

**Table 1.1**

Change of plasma concentration of a drugs with time after intravenous bolus administration of that drug expressed in terms of multiples of the plasma elimination half-life. The pattern of decline is applicable to all processes decribed by a half-life.

| Elapsed time after i.v. bolus injection expressed as multiples of the elimination half-life | Remaining plasma drug concentration expressed as a % of the initial concentration | Reduction of plasma concentration expressed as % of the original concentration |
|---|---|---|
| 0 | 100% | 0% |
| 1 | 50% | 50% |
| 2 | 25% | 75% |
| 3 | 12.5% | 87.5% |
| 4 | 6.25% | 93.75% |

Gerry continued. "When you look at the anesthetic chart of Mr. Terra, you see that his heart rate and blood pressure subsided to near normal levels 30 to 40 minutes after induction of anesthesia, a time about equivalent to three to four plasma elimination half-lives of epinephrine, and a time when about 90% of the excess epinephrine would have been eliminated from his plasma. This is a really nice clinical illustration of the concept of the plasma elimination half-life, because epinephrine is a hormone whose plasma concentration need only increase slightly above the normal range to cause tachycardia or increased blood pressure. So any increase of plasma epinephrine concentrations above normal levels must be eliminated before heart rate and blood pressure subside to normal levels. This is one of the reasons for that very frustrating phenomenon observed by all anesthesiologists—that some patients are only finally adequately under general anesthesia just when the surgeon finishes the operation. In addition, this example reveals that plasma elimination half-life has little to do with duration of action—plasma elimination half-life is only a description of how fast a drug or other substance is eliminated from the plasma. Is this all clear up till now?"

Bob nodded, "Yes."

"Now another interesting aspect about half-lives is the very fact of a half-life. Why is it that the speed of drug elimination out of plasma is described by an exponential decrease instead of a linear decrease? Make a guess as to why? I'll give a hint—the answer lies in body structure and function—not in the phantasmagoria of mathematics in many of the mind-bogglingly difficult books on pharmacokinetics."

"Is this recent research?" was Bob's response.

"Not at all—quite old in fact. The answer lies in the manner drugs are exchanged between plasma and extravascular tissues. The flow of blood through each organ and tissue of the body is a constant fraction of the cardiac output. This means that each second, minute, or hour, a certain volume of blood containing drugs at a certain concentration flows through each of the organs and tissues of the body. Diffusion is the principal mechanism by which drugs are exchanged between plasma and extravascular tissues. Now diffusion is an interesting process, because the speed with which molecules diffuse from one region to another is dependant on the difference in concentration between these regions. The higher the concentration gradient, the greater the speed of diffusion, and vice versa. This is why the change in plasma concentration of a drug passing through any organ or tissue is directly related to the plasma-to-tissue drug concentration gradient. The same is also true for drugs passing through drug eliminating organs. Drug elimination organs metabolize, or excrete drugs out of the body. Accordingly, drug concentrations in the tissues of these organs are lower than in the plasma, which is why drug molecules always diffuse out of the plasma into the tissues of these eliminating organs.

Let's look at an example of a very theoretical drug eliminated by the kidneys, whose entry into and out of kidney cells, tubules, and urine is determined solely by diffusion. Furthermore, let us assume this theoretical drug undergoes no metabolism or active transport within the kidneys. I mention this, because the elimination of some drugs by the kidneys is affected by active transport systems, as well as renal drug metabolism. So in our example, arterial blood enters the kidneys. Drug diffuses out of the renal capillaries into the tissues of the kidney, as well as being filtered into the glomerular filtrate, from where the drug is excreted in urine in its unchanged form. The result of this process is that renal vein plasma drug concentrations are lower than arterial plasma drug concentrations. Let us assume for the sake of this very theoretical example, that this drug undergoes very efficient renal excretion, so that the renal vein plasma drug concentration is 60% (= 0.6) of the renal arterial plasma drug concentration. The time for a drug to completely recirculate from one point in the human body back to that same point is about one minute (4). So the change of plasma concentration of this drug with time is shown by the list below."

- At time = 0 minutes, initial renal arterial plasma drug concentration = 100 units/liter, and renal vein plasma drug concentration = 100 x 0.6 = 60 units/liter.
- After one recirculation time = 1 minute, renal arterial plasma drug concentration = 60 units/liter, and renal vein plasma drug concentration = 60 x 0.6 = 36 units/liter.

- After two recirculation times = 2 minutes, renal arterial plasma drug concentration = 36 units/liter, and renal vein plasma drug concentration = 36 x 0.6 = 21.6 units/liter.
- After three recirculation times = 3 minutes, renal arterial plasma drug concentration = 21.6 units/liter, and renal vein plasma drug concentration = 21.6 x 0.6 = 12.96 units/liter.
- After four recirculation times = 4 minutes, renal arterial plasma drug concentration = 12.96 units/liter, and renal vein plasma drug concentration = 12.96 x 0.6 = 7.776 units/liter.
- And so on, and so on...

"Huh?... Mmmm..." began Bob, as if about to object to something.

"Yes, I know, I know," said Gerry quickly. "The systemic arterial concentrations of a drug are not necessarily the same as the renal venous concentrations of that same drug, because renal venous blood mixes with venous blood from the rest of the body, so reducing the effect of renal elimination on arterial drug concentrations. However, I always enjoy a bit of excessive physiological exaggeration for teaching purposes. In this very theoretical example, 100 - 60 = 40% of drug present in the plasma is removed from the circulation while passing through the kidney. This percentage removal of drug from the plasma is called the extraction ratio, and in this example the extraction ratio = 40% = 0.4. If you think more deeply, the extraction ratio for each organ can be translated into a plasma flow, a theoretical flow of plasma from which drug is totally eliminated, removed, or cleared from the plasma by an eliminating organ per unit time. For example, if the renal plasma flow in our example is 500 milliliters per minute, this means that each minute 500 x 0.4 = 200 milliliters of plasma is cleared of drug by the kidneys. This is the renal plasma clearance of this very theoretical drug. This same reasoning is applicable to every drug eliminating organ, as well as to the whole body. Now I'm going to stretch your mind with an equation expressing what I just said."

$$Cl = Q \times (1 - (C_{venous} / C_{arterial}))$$

- $Cl$ = plasma drug clearance of an organ, or the whole body, expressed as l/min.
- $Q$ = flow of plasma through an organ, or the whole body, expressed as l/min.
- $(C_{venous} / C_{arterial})$ = ratio of venous and arterial plasma drug concentrations.

Gerry continued, "This expresses all I just explained, and makes it possible to calculate how much drug is eliminated from the plasma per unit time."

$$E = Cl \times C_{arterial}$$

- $E$ = drug elimination rate from the plasma by an organ, or the whole body, expressed as mg/min.

"So," said Gerry, "these equations also make it evident that the concentration decrease of drug in plasma is exponential, because the rate of drug elimination decreases as the arterial plasma drug concentration decreases and vice versa. All this is applicable to the whole body, as well as to individual drug-eliminating organs. I'll spare you a detailed discussion of the mathematical properties of exponentials, because that is out of the scope of this book. If you're interested you can always look these things up in a book on basic mathematics."

Bob looked a little bemused, but the explanation was logical, and made matters much clearer to him. "That clears my thinking on this matter considerably," was his response. "Physiology does indeed seem to make pharmacokinetics more logical. I wonder why some people say physiology has nothing to do with pharmacokinetics?"

"I don't know why either," said Gerry at the same time as a nurse called over the intercom that Mr. Terra was welcome in the recovery room. "Aha, Bob I'll bring Mr. Terra to the recovery room. After that I'm off for a cup of coffee. Teaching is thirsty work. You can start with the next patient. You know what to do." With these words Gerry departed with Mr. Terra to the recovery room and a well-earned cup of coffee. The orderly brought the next patient inside. This was a man who was to undergo an inguinal hernia operation under spinal anesthesia.

Bob sighed. He also wanted a cup of coffee, but he knew his place within the hospital hierarchy. So he turned to the patient and began preparations for the spinal anesthetic.

# 2

## Asleep in ten seconds!!

Mrs. Dolore glared at Doctor Bob. "Ow! That hurt!"

"Sorry about that," replied Bob, "but you've got rolling veins, which means you have very thin skin and your veins roll away from the drip needle, so I had to prick three times before I finally got the drip in."

"But why do I need a drip? I didn't ask for it. I've come for a breast reduction operation. You're supposed to give me an anesthetic for the operation, not a drip. Doctor Dupuytren, my plastic surgeon, didn't tell me I needed a drip."

"There are two reasons why you need a drip," was Bob's patient answer. "You need a drip so we can administer anesthetic drugs without pricking you again, as well as to replace any fluids and blood you may lose during your breast reduction operation. Your drip is now in position, so I'm finished with the preparations for your anesthetic."

"Ohhh... So that's why I was asked whether I agreed to a blood transfusion if necessary. Even so, no one told me why I might need a blood transfusion. Why didn't anyone tell me all these things beforehand?"

"Mrs. Dolore, I know Doctor Dupuytren did tell you, because he noted it in your case notes, and I know that you were told about this in the anesthetic screening clinic, because it was noted there too. It's standard practice."

"Still, I can't remember anyone telling me these things," replied a disgruntled Mrs. Dolore.

Just then, as if he could sense the moment with some sort of sixth sense, Doctor Gerry walked into the operating theater. "Ah, I thought you might be ready by now Bob." He continued in a breezy tone, "Hello Mrs. Dolore, I'm Doctor Gerry, and I'm an anesthesiologist. Doctor Bob and I work together, and I see everything is ready for your operation. So let's get started. Bob, you stand at the head-end, and I'll inject the drugs."

The aura of authority, purpose, and competence radiating from Doctor Gerry silenced Mrs. Dolore, but only temporarily. She began again, "I've heard that general anesthetics act very quickly. My sister had the same operation last month, and she told me that she fell asleep within ten seconds. My niece also told me she couldn't even count to ten before she went under anesthesia. So I guess that means I'll also fall asleep before I can count to ten. When should I start counting?"

"Whenever you want," said Gerry. "Count all you like, but it'll still take at least 20 to 30 seconds before you're under." And he began to inject the contents of the opiate syringe into her drip, while at the same time saying to Bob, "We'll use the ASE technique with this lady."

"ASE technique?" asked Bob. "What do you mean by the ASE technique?"

"I'll explain it to you shortly. Just a moment while I inject the Propofol."

Mrs. Dolore began to look anxious, "Oh, I don't feel well at all. I feel dizzy and very strange in my head, and there's an awful taste on my tongue. Is everything alright? I am going to wake up from the anesthetic, aren't I?" She began to look about in an agitated fashion, attempted to withdraw her arm, and began to complain loudly, "My arm is cold, and it hurts. Ow, ow, ow, owwww...!", after which she fell asleep precisely 20 seconds after the Propofol syringe had been emptied. Her transition into unconsciousness was rewarded with a dose of muscle relaxant, subsequent to which Bob intubated her and commenced mechanical ventilation.

"Call the plastic surgeon! He can help positioning the patient for the operation HE wants to perform," called Gerry. "By the way Bob, Mrs. Dolore said something very interesting just before she fell asleep. She mentioned an awful taste on her tongue. That was the taste of Propofol. Put a drop of Propofol on your tongue, and you can taste what she tasted. Okay, the initial taste of Propofol isn't too bad, but the aftertaste is utterly revolting, and this is what all patients taste as blood containing Propofol courses through their tongues just before they fall asleep. Luckily most of them forget it. As regards your question—the ASE technique simply means All Syringes Empty. We used the ASE technique because this woman is extremely anxious and querulous. An anesthesiologist can't change these facts. Such people are only benefited by rapid general anesthesia to terminate their anxiety so they can be operated upon for the condition they came for. After all, these people don't come here for psychological advice from an anesthesiologist, they come for an operation. Interestingly enough, such people are seldom afraid of the operation, but are almost always terrified of general anesthesia. An unjustified fear, but still an ancient and deeply rooted human fear, and a fear eloquently expressed in a passage in the Holy Koran describing the almost instinctive attitude many people have regarding the relationship between sleep and death."

# Asleep in ten seconds!

*God takes away men's souls upon their death, and the souls of the living during their sleep. Those that are doomed He keeps with Him, and restores the others for a time ordained. (1)*

In the meantime, Doctor Gil Dupuytren the plastic surgeon had been duly called and entered the operating theater. He sighed upon seeing Gerry declaiming to Bob, immediately recognizing the signs of "that which was to come"—Gerry was about to teach his resident some arcane aspect of anesthesia. "Okay Gerry, get off your soapbox. Let's position the patient first. At least then I can start working."

Without any further banter or ado, Gil and Gerry rapidly positioned Mrs. Dolore in the standard half-sitting position for her breast reduction operation. Gil went off to scrub for the operation, while Bob and Gerry performed a last check that the patient's pressure points were free, checked the monitors, the ventilation, and double checked it all again. The automatic blood pressure meter repeatedly tried measuring the patient's blood pressure. So Gerry felt for pulsations over the superficial temporal artery in front of the Tragus. He felt nothing.

"Bob, give her 10 milligrams of Ephedrine. Now!" barked Gerry.

"But we haven't measured her blood pressure yet," was the response from Bob, "and 10 milligrams of Ephedrine is a bit much to administer without knowing what's going on."

"Bob, we do know what's going on. So give the Ephedrine, and I'll explain."

Bob administered 10 milligrams of Ephedrine. Shortly afterwards Gerry felt strong pulsations over the superficial temporal artery, and the automatic blood pressure meter measured a pressure of 105/65 mmHg.

19

Gerry relaxed and began. "Bob, anesthesia in a half-sitting, or sitting position is a bit like fainting in a telephone booth. If the blood pressure drops, not enough blood goes to the brain, and you get cerebral ischemia due to under-perfusion. Very well, some people say that blood pressure is unimportant, saying that the flow of blood is what is important. This is true, but these people forget one simple fact—in order for blood to flow through blood vessels, there must be sufficient blood pressure to drive the blood through the blood vessels. No blood pressure means no blood flow. Furthermore, we can't measure cerebral perfusion—we can only measure blood pressure. We know for certain that the cerebral perfusion of a person in a sitting position is normal at a reasonably normal blood pressure. Cerebral perfusion may also be reasonably normal at a reduced blood pressure too, but we don't know that for certain, which is why we have to choose safety first. A practical way of dealing with these facts is simply to feel the various pulses of the body. If you can't feel a pulse, then the blood pressure is too low and you do something about it. Here is a simple rule of thumb for blood pressure."

- You cannot feel pulsations over the radial artery below a systolic blood pressure of 40 to 50 mmHg.
- You cannot feel pulsations over the superficial temporal artery in front of the Tragus below a systolic blood pressure of 70 to 80 mmHg.

"The Tragus is about the same level as the brainstem. So if you can't feel pulsations over the superficial temporal arteries in front of the Tragus, then you know several things. No palpable pulsations means the patient is hypotensive, meaning that little blood is flowing through the superficial temporal artery at this level, which means that the same is occurring in the arteries inside the brain at this same level, meaning that the brainstem is possibly under-perfused. This requires action. So we administered 10 mg Ephedrine. But this is practical general medicine that has little to do with theoretical pharmacokinetics and pharmacodynamics. The response of this woman to her induction dose of Propofol illustrated two interesting kinetic and dynamic points: the speed with which she fell asleep, and the reason for her hypotension."

This last remark elicited an almost magical response from the surgical team. Restless murmurings and subdued moans arose from the other side of the sterile drapes separating anesthesiologists from surgeons. Those with acute hearing might have been able to distinguish soft moaning sounds that almost sounded like, "No, no... Make it stop, make it stop..." Dupuytren was also aroused to comment, "You really can wring a flood out of a damp rag Gerry." And with a weary sigh he added, "But go on, and on, and on with your lesson, we're all ears, we're agog, panting with anticipation to hear this new snippet of knowledge with which you want to enrich our dreary little lives." Upon which he indicated his total fascination by yawning in a loud and demonstrative manner.

Bob began to suspect this learning moment was not quite finished.

Gerry began. "Bob, can you tell me why it took so long for this woman to fall asleep? After all, I injected the Propofol directly into her bloodstream, so she should have slept within ten seconds like she imagined."

Bob thought a bit, and replied, "Has it something to do with the speed with which drugs are distributed throughout the central compartment?"

"Bob, just for this moment, forget all this mumbo-jumbo of half understood pharmacokinetic terms. Think like a doctor, a practical physiologist, a person who knows how the body is constructed and functions. Use practical common sense. Consider the following true statements."

- Hypnotic drugs do not cause people to sleep because their blood sleeps, but because these drugs diffuse out of capillaries into the tissues of the brainstem, inducing brainstem malfunction resulting in unconsciousness.
- Analgesic drugs do not relieve pain by an analgesic effect on blood cells, but because these drugs diffuse out of the capillaries into the tissues of those parts of the nervous system involved in the perception of pain, affecting these parts of the nervous system so as to reduce pain perception.
- Muscle relaxant drugs do not cause paralysis by paralyzing blood cells, but because they diffuse out of muscle capillaries into the tissues of muscles where they block transmission of nerve signals at neuromuscular junctions.

"This means that drugs must first arrive at the tissues where they act. So Bob, after injection of anesthetic drugs into blood vessels, how do they actually enter the tissues where they exert their effects?"

"Drugs injected into arteries or veins are transported by the flow of blood in blood vessels to all tissues of the body."

"Correct. Transport of drugs by the flow of blood in blood vessels explains the speed of onset of drugs, as well as the hypotension caused by induction doses of many hypnotic drugs. Can you tell me how?"

"Gerry, I was at a party until four o'clock his morning. So I'm not feeling altogether in top form. So could you make it a bit easier for me?"

"Hmmmm," came from Gerry, as he looked sternly and censoriously at Bob. "Very well, just for today, I'll let you have an easy time. Now just consider what happens when you inject Propofol or any other drug into a peripheral vein. Let's reconstruct what happened when I injected the Propofol into Mrs. Dolore's hand vein."

- I injected 200 mg Propofol into her hand vein over 10 seconds.
- Propofol is quite fat soluble, so it is a reasonable approximation to say that plasma and whole blood Propofol concentrations were equal.
- The injected Propofol mixed with the venous blood in her arm returning to her heart.
- The cardiac output of Mrs. Dolore would be about 5000 ml/min, which means her venous return is also 5000 ml/min, and 10 seconds of venous return = 5000 x 10/60 = 833 ml. Assume the Propofol mixed completely with this returning venous blood. This is a reasonable approximation.
- The Propofol then passed through her right heart. Assume the Propofol mixed completely with the blood in her right heart. The volume of blood in the right heart is about 120 ml, so the total volume of blood with which the Propofol mixed was now about = 833 + 120 = 953 ml.
- The Propofol then passed into her pulmonary blood vessels, mixing with her pulmonary blood volume, which is about 500 ml in most adults (2,3). Assume the Propofol mixed completely with her pulmonary blood volume. So the volume of blood in which the Propofol mixed was then = 953 + 500 = 1453 ml.
- The Propofol then passed through her left heart. Assume the Propofol mixed completely with the blood in her left heart. The volume of blood in the left heart is about 120 ml, so the total volume of blood with which the Propofol mixed was about =1453 + 120 =1573 ml.

- The Propofol induction dose was 200 mg. Accordingly, the initial concentration of Propofol in blood pumped by her heart into her aorta to subsequently enter her coronary arteries and arterial system was about = 200/1573 = 0.127 mg/ml = 127 mg/1.
- Now look at the concentration-effect relationships of some induction agents in this table (Table 2.1).

**Table 2.1**

| Drug | Average steady state plasma concentration causing hypnosis (mg/l) = brainstem concentration needed for hypnosis | Minimum plasma concentration causing myocardial depression (mg/l) |
|---|---|---|
| Thiopental | $10^4$ | $70^5$ |
| Methohexital | $3.4^6$ | $10^6$ |
| Etomidate | $0.21^7$ | $15^7$ |
| Propofol | $2^8$ | $10^9$ |

Gerry showed these figures, looked triumphant, and said, "This table makes two things immediately obvious."

- The initial concentration of Propofol in the arterial blood pumped out of the heart of Mrs. Dolore was 60 times that needed to cause sleep! Yet despite this, it could not cause her to sleep until it entered the capillaries of her brainstem, where it first had to diffuse into, and then affect the tissues of her brainstem before finally causing her to sleep. So it is not at all surprising she didn't fall asleep within the ten seconds she believed would happen, although once the Propofol arrived in her brainstem, onset of hypnosis was rapid because of the high blood Propofol concentration.

- Furthermore, the reason for her hypotension is also immediately obvious. The initial concentration of Propofol in the blood pumped through her aortic valve to enter her aorta, where it subsequently entered the ostia of her coronary arteries to perfuse her myocardium, was more than 12 times the concentration needed to cause myocardial depression! No wonder she was hypotensive. The cause of her hypotension was myocardial depression.

- In this situation, treatment of her hypotension with ephedrine was just as temporary as the cause. Ephedrine in doses up to 20 mg is a positive inotropic drug readily available to anesthesiologists. The use of Ephedrine, or other short acting inotropics for this purpose is much more logical than infusing vast volumes of fluids which remain a long time in the body, and which may subsequently cause heart failure.

"Practical experience teaches that 5 mg Ephedrine is simply too little for any significant effect in most adults, and 20 mg is excessive, which is why I asked for 10 mg. Sometimes post-induction hypotension causes significant myocardial ischemia in patients with coronary artery sclerosis, because myocardial perfusion in some of these patients is directly related to blood pressure. So in the elderly, or in those at risk of, or with known coronary artery disease, it is advisable to inject induction doses of hypnotic agents rather more slowly. Let's work out what would have happened had I injected the induction dose of Propofol into Mrs. Dolore more slowly than I did. Here it is again in list form."

- Inject 200 mg Propofol into a hand vein of Mrs. Dolore over 30 seconds instead of over 10 seconds.
- Propofol is quite fat soluble, so it is a reasonable approximation to say that plasma and whole blood Propofol concentrations are equal.
- The injected Propofol mixes with the venous blood in her arm returning to her heart. The cardiac output of Mrs. Dolore is about 5000 ml/min, which means a venous return of 5000 ml/min, and 30 seconds of venous return = 5000 x 30/60 = 2500 ml. Assume the Propofol mixed completely with this returning venous blood. This is a reasonable approximation.
- The right heart, left heart, and pulmonary blood volumes are the same as in our previous calculation, which is a volume = 120 + 120 + 500 = 740 ml. The total volume with which the Propofol mixes is then = 2500 + 740 = 3240 ml.
- The Propofol induction dose was 200 mg. Accordingly, the initial concentration of Propofol in blood pumped by her heart into her aorta to subsequently enter her coronary arteries and arterial system would have been = 200 / 3240 = 0.0617 mg/ml = 61.7 mg/1.
- This is a lower concentration than when the same dose is injected over 10 seconds. Accordingly, the degree of myocardial depression is less than with a rapid injection. And because the initial plasma concentration is still much higher than that needed in the brainstem to cause hypnosis, the Propofol will still diffuse sufficiently rapidly into the brainstem to cause a reasonably speedy hypnotic effect.

"So," continued Gerry, "as you see, slower injection rates mean lower peak concentrations, and therefore less myocardial depression, while at the same time still giving reasonably fast induction times. Only you need a lot more patience than with a rapid injection. One advantage of slower injection rates is that you can also induce hypnosis with a lower total dose of induction agent, with a resulting lower initial peak concentration causing an even lesser degree of myocardial depression. This is the safest method of administering intravenous induction agents to the elderly, to people with coronary vascular disease, as well as people with low cardiac outputs due to cardiac disease, or hypovolemia due to dehydration or hemorrhage."

"Oh, is that the reason why people say that American anesthesiologists killed more American military personnel with Thiopental after the Japanese bombing raid on Pearl Harbor on December 7, in 1941, than the Japanese killed with their bombs?"

"Oh Bob, you should really know better than to listen to gossip. That hoary old story about Thiopental at Pearl Harbor is a myth. There have been several studies of this story using the hospital admission data of the time, among which there is an excellent article by Bennetts in 1995 revealing this story to be a fable (10). True, a deliciously gruesome fable, but a fable nonetheless. After all, even at that time anesthesiologists were well aware of the dangers of administering Thiopental anesthesia to patients who were hypovolemic due to hemorrhage or dehydration, and they took due precautions. However there is an element of truth to this story, and it is fascinating to see what does happen when intravenous induction agents are used during hypovolemia due to all causes. So let's do a small calculation."

- Assume Mrs. Dolore is hypovolemic due to a massive hemorrhage.
- Propofol has the same effects on the heart and consciousness as Thiopental.

- Assume we are ignorant anesthesiologists, totally unaware of the risks of inducing anesthesia with normal doses of Propofol in hypovolemic patients. So we inject 200 mg Propofol into a hand vein of Mrs. Dolore over our usual 10 seconds. What will happen? This is where basic physiology and common sense gives wonderful insights.

- Propofol is quite fat soluble, so it is a reasonable approximation to say that plasma and whole blood Propofol concentrations are equal.

- The injected Propofol mixes with the venous blood in the arm of Mrs. Dolore, and returns to her heart. The cardiac output of Mrs. Dolore is normally 5000 ml/min, but severe hypovolemia has reduced it to 3000 ml/min, which also means a venous return of 3000 ml/min. Ten seconds of venous return = 3000 x 10/60 = 500 ml. Assume that Propofol mixes completely with this returning venous blood. This is a reasonable approximation.

- Right heart, left heart, and pulmonary blood volumes are also reduced due to hypovolemia, and are now = 100 + 100 + 400 = 600 ml. The total blood volume with which the Propofol initially mixes is then = 500 + 600 = 1100 ml.

- If we were so foolish in this situation to use our standard Propofol induction dose of 200 mg, the initial concentration of Propofol in blood pumped by her heart into her aorta to subsequently enter her coronary arteries and arterial system would be = 200/1100 = 0.181 mg/ml = 181 mg/1.

- This is a concentration far in excess of those required to cause loss of consciousness and myocardial depression (Table 2.1). The clinical effect on Mrs. Dolore would be severe cardiovascular shock and deep coma, possibly even death.

"Experimental studies show these effects do indeed occur when using intravenous induction agents such as Propofol and Thiopental (12,13). The lesson from these stories and this type of calculation is clear—when administering intravenous induction agents to hypovolemic patients, or patients with low cardiac outputs due to any of a multitude of causes, inject slowly, and use low doses. Furthermore, when you repeat these same calculations for other induction agents, one thing becomes immediately obvious—Etomidate is really the only induction agent that does not cause significant cardiac depression, a fact confirmed again and again by clinical practice. Now we've arrived at the question of how long it took for Mrs. Dolore to fall asleep. This is given by the well-known concept of circulation times. So Bob tell me about circulation times. What is a circulation time?"

Bob looked uncomfortable as well as hung-over. Even so, he tried squirming his way out of giving an answer that would reveal his ignorance. "Isn't circulation time a rather old-fashioned concept? No-one ever uses it."

"Well Bob, have I got news for you. Circulation times are far from dead. They are very much alive—living in this book, this lesson, throughout all practical anesthetic practice, as well as in high flying jetliners. They are a very practical method of timing the speeds with which substances injected at one point in the body arrive at another point. Just look at the following circulation times in this table (Table 2.2)."

They looked at the table while Gerry continued, "This table shows it takes about 13 to 20 seconds for a drug injected in the arm to arrive at the brain. This is why I knew Mrs. Dolore simply could not fall asleep before 20 seconds had passed. It takes a period equivalent to one arm-brain circulation time before any induction agent arrives in the capillaries of the brainstem. Only then, can an anesthetic induction agent begin to diffuse from the plasma into the tissues of the brainstem and induce loss of consciousness. Most clinically employed anesthetic induction agents are administered at relatively high doses, so the initial peak plasma concentrations are high enough to induce sleep within seconds after passing through brainstem capillaries. This is why induction of hypnosis never occurs precisely after one arm-brain circulation time, but always a few seconds afterwards. Accordingly, it was simply impossible for Mrs. Dolore to fall asleep within 10 seconds. All these things explain what we observed happening to this woman during induction of anesthesia."

**Table 2.2**

Some circulation times (11)

| From where to where | Time (seconds) |
| --- | --- |
| Arm vein to lung | 5-8 |
| Arm vein to left ventricle | 6-8 |
| Arm vein to tongue | 12-15 |
| Arm vein to brain | 13-20 |
| Foot vein to tongue | 37-47 |
| Right heart to ear | 8 |
| Arm to foot | 21-35 |

"Okeeee....," said Bob, "that certainly makes the reason for induction times and clinical effects clearer to me. But how could circulation times be of any relevance in high flying jetliners?"

"Bob, have you ever gone anywhere, or flown to your holiday destination in a passenger jetliner?"

"Yes."

"Most modern jetliners cruise at an altitude of about 11,000 meters. This necessitates pressurizing the cabin to a much lower altitude, because air at 11,000 meters altitude contains too little oxygen to sustain human life. Just before take-off, you always get the obligatory talk about emergency procedures. One part of these emergency instructions covers what to do if the cabin suddenly decompresses. This instruction consists of informing people to put on the oxygen masks that automatically drop down from the ceiling upon sudden cabin decompression. All those who understand are clearly instructed to put on their oxygen masks first, and only after they have put on their oxygen masks, to help children or other less able people with their masks. You may think this is a strange instruction, as well as being totally against all natural instincts and normal behavior. After all, your natural instinct is to save the children first, because adults are older and less valuable than children. Furthermore, as regards those adults with difficulty putting on their masks, many altruistic people first try to aid those less able than themselves."

"Always wondered about that myself," interrupted Dupuytren. "But I finally realized this rule must have been devised for the situation of a planeload of plastic surgeons. After all, plastic surgeons are superior beings who are certainly more valuable than lesser mortals and children."

Gerry ignored these comments from the peanut-gallery. He continued. "If an airplane cabin suddenly decompresses at 11,000 meters altitude, just about all the air in the lungs is sucked out, and the remaining oxygen pressure in the lungs is too low to sustain consciousness and life. From that moment on, no significant amounts of oxygen combine with the hemoglobin in blood passing through the lungs. From that time onwards all the blood pumped by the heart to the rest of the body is severely oxygen-depleted. Eventually this severely oxygen-depleted blood reaches the brainstem, and a few seconds later oxygen starvation causes brainstem malfunction manifesting as unconsciousness. Now a circulation time is the time it takes blood to go from one part of the body to another, and these times give us part of the answer to how long it takes humans to lose consciousness due to sudden decompression at an altitude of 11,000 meters, or higher. The relevant circulation time here is the right heart-to-ear circulation time, which is about eight seconds in the average adult. The brainstem is about the same distance from the heart as the ear, which means that oxygen-depleted blood will start arriving in the brainstems of passengers in such an unlucky jetliner about eight seconds after decompression. Sudden cessation of blood flow to the head during cardiac arrest is a similar situation to that occurring when blood flowing through the head no longer contains adequate amounts of oxygen. The time to loss of consciousness after sudden cessation of blood flow to the head resulting from cardiac arrest is between 5 to 20 seconds (14). Add these times to the right heart to ear circulation time, and you've calculated that loss of consciousness will occur about 13 to 28 seconds after sudden cabin decompression at high altitudes. American air force studies in the 1950's confirm these times (15). This is enough time for most adults—although I have my doubts about some surgeons—to understand what is going on, and quickly put on an oxygen mask. But if the adults first try to put oxygen masks onto their panicked and screaming offspring, these adults will all be unconscious before finally succeeding, and neither these adults, nor their children will receive any oxygen. So adults capable of doing so must put on their masks first, after which they can devote their time to helping their children, or aiding others less able to manage correct positioning of their oxygen masks. This is a beautifully logical application of the old-fashioned circulation times you thought had no current application."

Bob was stunned into silence by the simple beauty of this reasoning, but not Dupuytren, who was a real Philistine when it came to elegant scientific explanations. His voice rose above the sterile drapes, "Hey Gerry, I really learned lot today. Fantastic! You must be worn out after all that talking. Shouldn't you be resting and doing things anesthesiologists normally do, like drinking coffee, or whatever?"

"Well Bob, I guess this is one of those few moments that a surgeon is right about an exclusively anesthesiological matter. This is enough teaching for one day. So I'm off for a cup of coffee. Tell me when the operation is finally finished." And Gerry strolled out of the operating theater in the direction of the coffee room, leaving Bob a lesson wiser to continue the anesthetic for the operation."

# 3

# Compartmentalized & distributed

"Looks like we've got a problem with an anatomical variation here," said Doctor Hawley Crippen in an agitated tone redolent of increasing desperation, as he applied the diathermy at maximum power to yet another piece of bleeding tissue deep in the pelvis of a woman undergoing a hysterectomy. The scrub nurse turned her head aside to avoid the clouds of acrid smoke rising from the depths of the pelvis, while rolling her eyes upwards as if beseeching celestial assistance to stop the bleeding. But the bleeding did not stop, so she handed Crippen yet another haemostatic clamp. Bob and Gerry looked at each other. They knew the signs. This gynecologist had already recited the complete litany of standard complaints during the last hour, such as: "The light isn't any good. This scalpel is blunt. The blades of these scissors don't close properly. The patient isn't relaxed. These retractors have the wrong curve. You aren't using the retractor correctly! The anesthetic is too deep." Crippen was going to take a very long time to finish this hysterectomy. Luckily Mrs. Elmore was the last patient on his operating list, and luckily for her, she was under general anesthesia.

Gerry walked around the operating table, assessed the amount of blood on the drapes and floor, as well as checking the volume of blood in the suction pots. Finally, he looked critically into the abdominal wound, saw a sight evoking imagery of a smoldering middle ages plague pit, sighed loudly and wearily, and looked upwards as if also seeking succor from the heavens. But just as with the scrub nurse, the much-desired heavenly intervention failed to arrive. He turned to Bob, and said in a voice clearly able to be heard by Crippen, "Well Bob, it looks like we have some time on our hands, so it's time to stretch your mind. Let's talk about intravenous anesthetic induction agents. We used 250 mg Thiopental to induce anesthesia in Mrs. Elmore. There is nothing unusual about this woman, except that she enjoys smoking about 20 cigarettes, as well as drinking at least three glasses of wine a day. There was also nothing unusual about her reaction to this perfectly standard induction dose. So if we administered no other drugs, how long would you expect her to remain asleep with this dose of Thiopental?"

"About ten minutes," replied Bob, "and perhaps even less, because she drinks three glasses of wine a day, so her liver will metabolize Thiopental more rapidly than that of a person who doesn't drink as much. Accordingly she will eliminate Thiopental quicker and wake up more rapidly than normal." Bob was quite pleased with this answer. It was physiologically oriented, and really did correspond with reality, because smoking cigarettes and drinking alcohol really do induce drug metabolizing liver enzymes. This explanation was what he had heard from everyone else, and could not fail to satisfy Gerry's lust for physiologically oriented answers.

Gerry appeared to be in pain, demonstratively clutched the anesthetic machine for support, and groaned, "Ohhhh, just as I was beginning to think the light of understanding was beginning to dawn in your mind, you start uttering pseudo-physiological gibberish you must have heard from other people. Sadly, this is a popular delusion, even among people who should know better." Gerry assumed his lesson-giving stance. "Now Bob, you are quite correct, ten minutes to waking up after such a dose of Thiopental is perfectly normal for just about all adults. But as for the rest of your answer—what you said is true enough, but totally irrelevant in this context. After all, what you are actually telling me with your answer is that this woman, and all other people awaken after about ten minutes because of rapid elimination of Thiopental from their bodies. If you believe that, then you probably still believe in pixies, and that a good flogging together with exorcism of demons is a modern treatment for epilepsy. I see I'm going to have to do some work to correct this delusion. So let's begin with the basics. Tell me, what is the plasma elimination half-life of Thiopental? This plasma elimination half-life is no fantasy, but a product of real measurements of real Thiopental plasma concentrations made in real people. Look it up if you want (Appendix)."

Bob began to look uncertain, hauled his notebook out of his pocket, quickly leafed through to the pharmacokinetic datasheet, and replied, "Er, about 13 hours..."

"Well Bob, as you know, Thiopental is transported by the blood to the brainstem, where it diffuses out of the capillaries into the tissues of the brainstem to induce unconsciousness. The brainstem does not metabolize Thiopental, which means that brainstem tissue Thiopental concentration is determined by the plasma Thiopental concentration, because it is blood that transports Thiopental to and from the brainstem. Now, the Thiopental elimination half-life you just told me is the plasma elimination half-life, and not the half-life for elimination of Thiopental from the body (Chapters 1 and 3). So Bob, you're actually trying to tell me that people wake up about ten minutes after receiving a perfectly normal induction dose of Thiopental because rapid hepatic metabolism reduces the plasma concentration of Thiopental to a level below that needed to keep them asleep. We're talking here about a drug with a plasma elimination half-life of 13 hours! How much Thiopental do you think this patient, or any other patient for that matter, will have eliminated from their plasma after ten minutes?"

"Not much."

"Quite right. Practically nothing. Within the time this woman, or any other patient awakens after an induction dose of an intravenous anesthetic induction agent, the entire drug dose is still present within the body. Very little, to no plasma elimination will have occurred within ten minutes."

"Then I guess people awaken for some other reason'

"Very good Bob, it seems you're learnt your lesson about plasma elimination half-lives well. So why do you think people wake up so rapidly after Thiopental? Look at your table of kinetic and dynamic data again (Appendix)."

Bob looked in his notebook again, and thought a few seconds before replying, "I guess it must be related to the plasma distribution half-life of Thiopental. After all that's very short, only about 3.3 minutes. If I apply the same reasoning to the plasma distribution half-life as we did with the plasma elimination half-life (Table 1.1), then the process of distribution will be almost complete (87.5% complete), after three plasma distribution half-lives = 3 x 3.3 = 9.9 minutes, which is about ten minutes. So this means people awaken ten minutes after an induction dose of Thiopental because distribution of this drug throughout the body is complete."

"You're getting quite good at this," was Gerry's answer. "You're quite correct. People wake up after a hypnotic dose of an induction agent because of distribution of drug throughout the body. But what do you mean by distribution? How do you see the relationship between distribution, the falling asleep, the awakening of the patient, and plasma elimination of Thiopental in this case, and all other drugs in general?"

"All I see are these complicated formulae and parameters in most books, and the relationship of these to physiology is not all that obvious to me. But I'm sure you would love to explain it to me."

"Don't know about that last bit, but I'll explain it anyway. First the basics," upon which Gerry expounded the following list.

- Consider what happens when a single intravenous bolus of a drug is administered. The injected drug mixes with the venous blood returning to the heart, and eventually the heart pumps this blood into the aorta, which conducts it to the arteries going to each organ and tissue of the body.
- Some organs, such as the brain, liver, and kidneys receive a high percentage of the cardiac output. Other organs such as muscles, intestines, and skin receive a lower percentage of the cardiac output. And others, such as fat and bone receive an even lower percentage of the cardiac output (Table 3.1).
- This means that much of an injected dose of a drug will initially diffuse into the tissues of organs with a high blood flow, such as the brain, kidneys, and liver. However, at the same time the circulation also transports drug into the capillary beds of the very much larger mass of organs with a lower blood flow, and drug also diffuses into the tissues of these organs.
- The result of all this is that drug concentrations are initially higher in the tissues of organs with a high blood flow such as brain, liver, and kidneys, than in the very much larger bulk of tissues with a lower blood flow, such as skin, muscle, bones, and fat.
- Diffusion of drug into the much larger mass of lower blood flow tissues continues. Eventually the plasma concentrations of drug in the blood drop below those in tis-

sues with a high blood flow, such as the brain. The result is that drug diffuses out of the tissues of the brain, and all other organs with a high blood flow back into the circulation. Continuing transportation of drug by the circulation to all tissues of the body means that drug diffuses into these organs and tissues, so reducing plasma drug concentrations even further. In the case of Thiopental, the plasma Thiopental concentration eventually falls below that required to induce, or to sustain unconsciousness.

- This process is called distribution, and as you correctly said or guessed, the speed of this distribution is given by the distribution half-life.

"This explains why Mrs. Elmore and all other people wake up so quickly after a normal induction dose of Thiopental, as well as after normal doses of all other intravenous induction agents. Is this clear?" asked Gerry.

"Very," was the curt response.

"Don't think you're going to get away this easily," said Gerry. "Now it's time to introduce a few concepts vital to your pharmacokinetic and pharmacodynamic development."

"Uh oh," thought Bob. "This could turn out to be a long teaching session. And I'm still not quite awake after the party last night." But he knew how to play this game, so he said aloud, "Do you mean the relationship between pharmacokinetics, pharmacodynamics, and physiology?"

"Absolutely. These are core concepts integrating the seemingly different aspects of physiology, pharmacokinetics, and pharmacodynamics. Practical application of these basic ideas will give you the ability to use existing drugs much better than before, as well as the ability to predict the behavior of new drugs. So let's begin."

**Table 3.1**

Organ weight and blood flow

| Organ | Organ blood flow (ml/100 g/min) | Organ weight (% body weight) |
|---|---|---|
| Kidneys | 340 | 0.5 |
| Liver | 100 | 2 |
| Heart | 69 | 0.4 |
| Brain | 54 | 2.3 |
| Skeletal muscle | 10-12 | 43 |
| Skin | 11 | 7 |
| Adipose tissue | 2-7 | 16-36 |

A harried bleating rose from the other side of the sterile drape separating anesthesia territory from that of the gynecology, "I want some silence in MY operating theater." Crippen continued, "Get out, or be quiet. I'm trying to perform a difficult operation, and your cackling is so distracting that I can't work properly."

Gerry looked over the sterile sheet into gynecology territory and saw the eyes of one scrub nurse rolling, while the other nurse looked desperately above. But as before, no angelic forms descended from the heavens to miraculously cure the patient and whisk them all away from this place. Mrs Elmore, Doctor Crippen, and the scrub nurses would have to do it together with some help from the anesthesiologist. Gerry fleetingly wondered if you could get periorbital muscle cramps or spasms from excessive eyeball rolling as he exclaimed, "What a good idea Hawley! It's time to indulge my caffeine addiction after working so hard. I'm off to relax and drink a delicious cup of coffee. So I'll leave you to get on with it. Bob, ask Bert to take over here for a while, and join me in the coffee room. We'll continue this lesson there."

Shortly afterwards, Bob joined Gerry in the otherwise empty coffee room. After taking a sip of black coffee, Gerry pulled a scrap of paper out of a pocket, found a pen, and began talking. "After you inject a single dose of a drug into the body, the blood transports it to all parts of the body where it diffuses into the tissues and organs of all parts of the body. At the same time, some of the organs and tissues into which the injected drug diffuses remove the drug from the body, either by excretion of the un-changed drug, or by metabolism of the drug. This latter is the process of elimination. When you look at it like this, you can say the volume of the body into which the drug is injected and is eliminated is a single volume. This is called a one-compartment model, and can be drawn as in Figure 3.1. In this model the drug is distributed throughout the distribution volume labeled $V_d$ The equation describing the plasma drug concentration with time after intravenous injection of a single bolus dose of a drug into the body is given below."

$$C = Be^{-\beta t}$$

- $C$ = plasma drug concentration.
- $B$ = a drug-specific constant.
- $e$ = a transcendental mathematical constant with the value 2.718.
- $t$ = elapsed time after drug administration.
- $\beta$ = a drug-specific constant whose value is given by: $\beta = 0.693/t_{1/2\beta}$ , where $t_{1/2\beta}$ = plasma elimination half-life of the drug.

# One Compartment

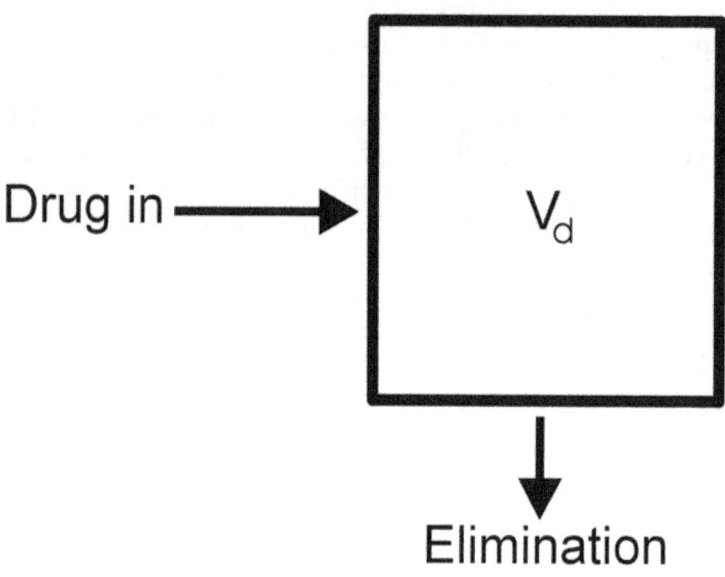

Figure 3.1: A single compartment pharmacokinetic model where the administered drug theoretically mixes within one compartment and is eliminated from that same compartment.

"All these things mean that the speed with which the plasma drug concentration declines is solely determined by the rate of elimination of the drug from the plasma, in this case the plasma elimination half-life. Do you follow me Bob?"

Bob looked vacantly at the equation. His only comment was, "Er...yes."

"I knew you would be excited. I always think it's wonderful how natural logarithms and transcendental numbers describe so many aspects of body function. Something mystical there. Makes you think there is some sort of grand order in the universe. So let's proceed further."

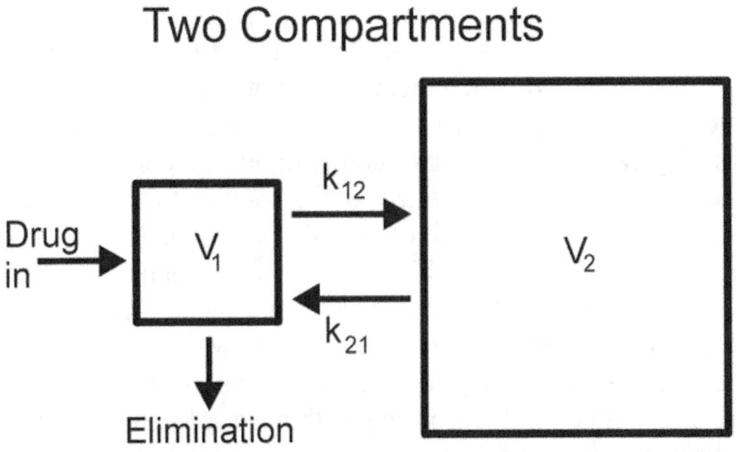

# Two Compartments

Figure 3.2: A two-compartment pharmacokinetic model where drug enters into, and is eliminated from a central compartment, as well as distributing into, and out of a second parallel peripheral compartment.

Totally disregarding the ever more vacant expression on the face of Bob, Gerry proceeded further. "As you know, the human body is not homogenous, so you must have realized immediately that this single compartment model of drug distribution is woefully inadequate. After all, the circulation transports intravenously administered drugs to body tissues of enormously variable composition. Some organs and tissues are mainly composed of fat, there is muscle tissue, there are all sorts of different organs with very diverse compositions, there are bones, and there is a lot of gooey stuff inside and between all these things. In addition to differences between the compositions of different tissues, the blood flow per unit weight of each tissue and organ also differs considerably (Table 3.1). This latter explains why an intravenously administered drug initially mainly diffuses into organs with higher blood flows before a significant amount of the drug diffuses into the tissues of organs with lower blood flows. Accordingly, you can conceive of drugs being distributed to higher and lower blood flow tissues, or two functional compartments. This is the physiological basis of the two-compartment model of drug pharmacokinetics. One compartment is the so-called central compartment, which is composed of blood, perivascular extracellular space, and the tissues of high blood flow organs. The second compartment is called the peripheral, or deep compartment, and comprises the larger part of the body mass which is composed of lower blood flow organs and tissues. This can be drawn schematically as in Figure 3.2. According to this two-compartment model, the plasma drug concentration decreases according to the equation below after intravenous injection of a single bolus dose of a drug. However, the pharmacokinetic properties of many anesthetic drugs are often better described with models using more than two compartments, such as the popular three-compartment model shown by figure 3.3. Models with even more compartments exist, but their clinical relevance is somewhat dubious."

$$C = Ae^{-\alpha t} + Be^{-\beta t}$$

- C = plasma drug concentration.
- A = a drug-specific constant.
- B = a drug-specific constant.
- e = a transcendental mathematical constant with the value 2.718.
- t = elapsed time after drug administration,

- $\alpha$ = a drug-specific constant whose value is given by: $\alpha = 0.693/t_{1/2\alpha}$, where $t_{1/2\alpha}$ = the plasma distribution half-life of the drug.
- $\beta$ = a drug-specific constant whose value is given by: $\beta = 0.693/t_{1/2\beta}$, where $t_{1/2\beta}$ = plasma elimination half-life of the drug.

# Three Compartments

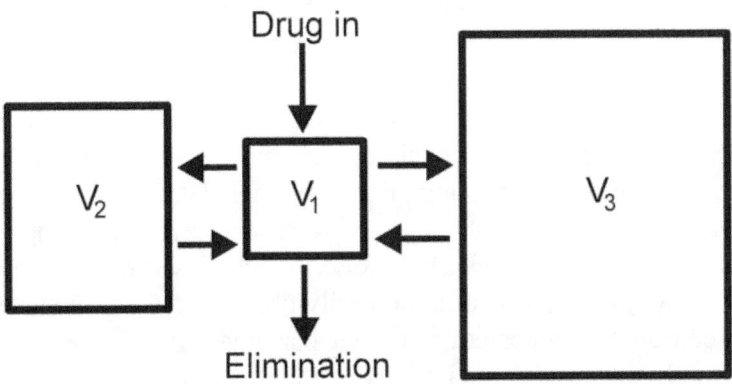

Figure 3.3: The most common form of a 3-compartment pharmacokinetic model. Drug enters into, and is eliminated from a central compartment ($C_1$), while at the same time distributing into, and out of two parallel peripheral compartments. One of these peripheral compartments ($C_2$) has an intermediate rate of exchange with the central compartment. The third, or deep peripheral compartment ($C_3$) has a much slower rate of drug exchange with the central compartment.

By now it was evident that a cup of strong coffee had not been sufficient to arouse Bob. This was totally lost on Gerry, who regarded Bob's vacant staring at these models and equations as proof he was almost cataplexic with excitement. Bob made an almost superhuman effort to arouse himself to ask a pertinent question. "Why don't we simply use a physiological mathematical model instead of all these complicated equations and unphysiological models which don't really seem to relate all that well to the structure and function of the body?"

"To begin with, a physiological model requires a set of constants for each organ and tissue of the body. Obtaining such data for each drug means serial biopsies of each and every organ and tissue in the body after administration of a drug. This would have to be done for several persons for each drug for which we want to obtain data. However, there are surprisingly few people willing to subject themselves to being biopsied to death for the sake of pharmacokinetic data. Physiological models have been constructed using deficient animal tissue drug data, but because of these deficient data they are no more accurate than empirical multi-compartment pharmacokinetic models based only on blood data. After all, blood is a tissue easily obtained from humans, and you can do that repeatedly without harming the volunteers from whom pharmacokinetic data are obtained. This is why all pharmacokinetic data in current use are based upon data obtained from serial blood sampling.

Bob barely concealed a yawn, and interrupted, "Thrilling stuff, but what is the clinical relevance to me? Are these equations and concepts useful in my clinical practice?"

"Actually, all these multicompartment equations are totally useless in clinical practice. They are too complex to be useful, and no-one carries a pocket computer to calculate drug doses and regimens while administering anesthesia, because practical clinical experience always yields a better result. However, the concepts associated with these models and parameters yield extraordinarily useful practical insights. These insights make drug administration predictable, give you understanding of how you use current drugs, how you can use them in new ways, how you can solve clinical problems related to drug use, as well as how you can use new drugs with which you have no experience at all. I'll explain how by beginning with the basics. To begin with, it is certainly true that the three-compartment model is a more accurate mathematical model for many anesthetic drugs, but as I said, is too complex for simple calculations. So I will restrict myself to the two-compartment model, which while not as accurate as the three-compartment model, is a model that is very easy to use without recourse to complicated calculations. Furthermore, it is a model providing valuable clinical insights, and calculations based on this model yield usable results that are sufficiently accurate for clinical practice. Here are the relevant parameters for the two compartment pharmacokinetic model."

- $V_1$ or $V_c$ = central compartment volume in liters per kilogram body weight. I will use liters per kilogram body weight as the unit of volume in this book.
- $V_2$ = peripheral compartment volume, otherwise also known as the deep compartment volume, in liters per kilogram body weight.
- $V_d$ = total volume of distribution in liters per kilogram body weight = $V_1 + V_2$. There are actually several other definitions of $V_d$ too, but while these are relevant when considering detailed mathematical analysis, they are irrelevant in this book because no precise calculations are made. The interested reader is advised to consult relevant textbooks on pharmacokinetics.
- Distribution of drugs between higher flow and lower flow tissues is a reasonably rapid process. This process of distribution is characterized by a rapid decline of plasma drug concentrations in the period immediately after intra-

venous bolus administration. This period is called the distribution phase (Figure 3.4). The speed with which this process of distribution of drug throughout the body occurs is expressed by the plasma distribution half-life.

- $t_{1/2\alpha}$ = plasma distribution half-life in minutes. Throughout the rest of this book, I will use the term distribution half-life to actually mean the plasma distribution half-life. This is standard terminology for all pharmacokinetic data of anesthetic drugs.

- After the process of distribution slows down, a second phase characterized by a slower decline in plasma drug concentration becomes evident. This slower rate of decline of plasma drug concentration is due to diffusion of drug into volumes of tissue with a low blood flow, as well as being due to metabolism and elimination of the drug from the body. It is should be noted that these processes also begin immediately after drug administration, but their effects on the plasma drug concentration only become evident after the distribution phase is complete. This phase is called the elimination phase (Figure 3.4). Even so, the term elimination phase only means that drug is eliminated from the plasma—it does not mean that drug is eliminated from the body. The speed with which this process of drug elimination from the plasma occurs is given by the plasma elimination half-life.

- $t_{1/2\beta}$ = plasma elimination half-life in minutes. Throughout the rest of this book, I will use the term elimination half-life to actually mean the plasma elimination half-life. This is standard terminology for all pharmacokinetic data of anesthetic drugs. Again, it cannot be emphasized enough that the elimination half-life is not necessarily the speed with which a drug is eliminated from the body—it only

describes the rate of change of plasma drug concentration during the elimination phase.
- D = drug dose in milligrams per kilogram body weight.
- C = plasma drug concentration in milligrams/liter.
- 2-compartment pharmacokinetic data for many anesthetic drugs are listed in the appendix.

"So let's apply 2-compartment pharmacokinetic principles to answer the question I asked earlier. How long will it take for Mrs. Elmore to awaken after a normal 250 mg intravenous dose of Thiopental if nothing is done to keep her asleep? Look up the relevant parameters for me and we'll put them in a list (see data in Appendix)." Without any further ado, Gerry and Bob made the following list.

- Body weight of Mrs. Elmore = 50 kg.
- Dose of Thiopental = 250 mg = 5 mg/kg body weight.
- Thiopental is very fat-soluble which is why you can say that plasma and blood Thiopental concentrations are approximately equal.
- Volume of blood with which drug mixes before emerging into her aorta after the first passage through her heart =1.5 liters (see Chapter 2).
- $V_c$ = 0.128 l/kg.
- $V_d$ = 3.5 l/kg.
- $t_{1/2\alpha}$ = 3.3 min.
- $t_{1/2\beta}$ = 781 min = 13 hours.
- Plasma Thiopental concentration causing myocardial depression = 70 mg/1 (Table 2.1).
- Plasma Thiopental concentration causing hypnosis =10 mg/1 (Table 2.1).

Bob looked at the list of pharmacokinetic parameters and began to look dissatisfied, unhappy even. He interrupted. "There's something wrong with the volume of distribution. The $V_d$ in this list is 3.5 l/kg. Now I know the specific gravity of the human body is almost equal to one kilogram per liter body volume (actually somewhere between 0.99 to 1.07 kg/1), which is why people can float more easily in seawater (specific gravity 1.03 kg/1), than in fresh water (specific gravity 1.0 kg/1). So a volume of distribution like this means that for each kilogram or liter of body volume, Thiopental occupies a volume of 3.5 liters! This can't be right! When I look at the tables of pharmacokinetic data in the appendix, I also see many other ridiculously improbable volumes of distribution. You talk about the mathematical phantasmagoria of pharmacokinetics—well this looks like a good example. How can such volumes be possible?"

"Bob, I'm a doctor, and I'm your mentor. Would I lie to you? So believe me when I say these volumes are true. I'll explain why very shortly. In the meantime, suspend your disbelief, and we can start doing some calculations for Mrs. Elmore," said Gerry, upon which he proceeded to make the following list.

- The volume of blood with which Thiopental mixes on the first passage through the heart and lungs is about 1.5 liters (Chapter 2). So Mrs. Elmore's initial aortic blood Thiopental concentration based upon the volume of blood with which drugs mix during their first passage through the heart and lungs = 250/1.5 = 167 mg/1. However, this is our physiologically based calculation.
- Based on 2-compartment pharmacokinetic data, the initial plasma Thiopental concentration in the $V_c$ of Mrs. Elmore before distribution begins = Dose/$V_c$ = 5/0.128 = 39 mg/1.

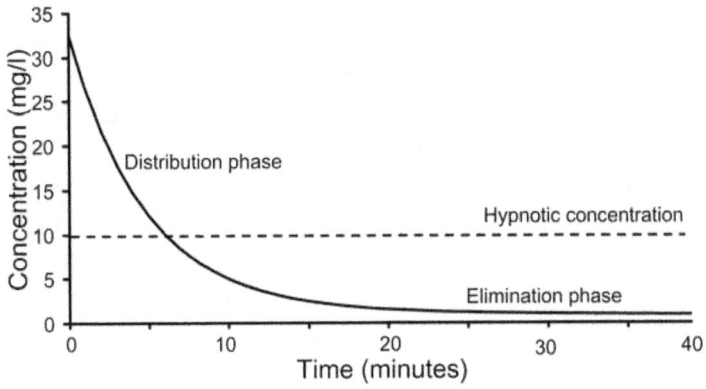

Figure 3.4: Plasma concentration-time curve of a 250 mg dose of Thiopental administered to an average adult. Note the initial rapid decline in plasma concentration due to drug distribution throughout the body, (distribution phase), and the subsequent slower decline of plasma drug concentration due to further distribution of drug within the body, as well as elimination, (elimination phase). The hypnotic concentration is the average plasma Thiopental concentration at which most people awaken.

Gerry continued, "These two initial Thiopental plasma concentrations are quite different. Even so, both initial plasma Thiopental concentrations describe why Mrs. Elmore fell asleep rapidly. But only the physiologically based model really explains the myocardial depression we also observed. Let's continue our exercise."

- Assuming no plasma drug elimination at ten minutes after Thiopental injection, then Mrs. Elmore's plasma Thiopental concentration after complete distribution = Dose/$V_d$ = 5/3.5 = 1.43 mg/l. This is a reasonable assumption because is evident from the relationship between the distribution and elimination half-lives, that practically no Thiopental will have been eliminated from her plasma before completion of distribution.

- So after complete distribution throughout the volume of distribution, blood Thiopental concentration will have fallen far below that which is needed to cause hypnosis or myocardial depression. Therefore metabolism plays no role in awakening after a single induction dose of Thiopental. Instead, distribution of the drug throughout the body is the reason a person awakens after an induction dose of Thiopental.

Gerry continued. "The following list illustrates this point."

- After one distribution half-life = 3.3 minutes, plasma Thiopental concentration will have fallen from 39 mg/1 to about 20 mg/1.
- After two distribution half-lives = 6.6 minutes, plasma Thiopental concentration will have fallen from 20 mg/1 to about 10 mg/1.
- Accordingly it will take somewhere between two and three distribution half-lives for a person to awaken after such a dose of Thiopental, i.e. somewhere between 6.6 and 10 minutes.
- Figure 3.4 shows the calculated plasma Thiopental concentrations after intravenous bolus administration of 250 mg to an average patient such as Mrs. Elmore. This figure also shows the distribution and elimination phases.

"This is what I mean by insights," said Gerry. "When used in this manner, these parameters provide invaluable insights. This example is a beautiful demonstration of the fact that the mechanism of termination of the hypnotic action of Thiopental is distribution, and not metabolism as popular superstition would have it. Think about it. You can perform this same type of calculation for all anesthetic induction agents and gain similar, or other valuable insights."

"I must admit this is certainly a useful method," was Bobs grudging reply. "I'll try it out on the other induction agents."

"You do that. But there is one last physiological insight I want to leave you with—the relationship of pharmacokinetic volumes to real physiological volumes. You were wondering how the pharmacokinetic volumes of some drugs could be larger than the volume of the body, or the other fluid compartment volumes of the body (Table 3.2). To begin with, there is one important consideration to keep in mind when looking at pharmacokinetic parameters of anesthetic drugs—unless otherwise stated, they are all based upon measurements of plasma drug concentrations. Looked at very simply, a pharmacokinetic volume is measured by administering a known dose of a drug, and then measuring its concentration in the volume into which it is administered. The drug concentration is given by the relationship below."

**Concentration = Dose / Volume**

Gerry continued, "Now in the case of measurements performed for pharmacokinetic purposes, we know the drug dose, and we can measure the drug concentration. This means that the unknown pharmacokinetic volume is given by the following relationship."

**Volume = Dose / Concentration**

"Are you following me so far Bob?" asked Gerry.
"Yes, even though you seem to be taking your time about it."

"First crawl then walk young man. Now, here it comes. Into which fluid do we administer anesthetic drugs, and in which fluid do we measure drug concentration?"

"We administer drugs intravenously, meaning we administer them into blood. As regards drug concentrations, you've repeatedly told me that all pharmacokinetic drug concentrations are plasma drug concentrations. So the drug concentrations measured for pharmacokinetic purposes are plasma drug concentrations," replied Bob.

**Table 3.2**

Volumes of different body compartments in "average" adults

| Fluid compartment | Men (l/kg) | Women (l/kg) |
|---|---|---|
| Total Body Water | 0.55 | 0.50 |
| Extracellular Fluid Volume | 0.25 | 0.20 |
| Interstitial Fluid Volume | 0.175 | 0.13 |
| Blood Volume | 0.075 | 0.07 |
| Plasma Volume | 0.045 | 0.04 |

"Very good Bob. You've learned that lesson well. And there you have the reason for these sometimes improbably large pharmacokinetic volumes. For example, if a drug is enormously fat soluble, and practically insoluble in something as watery as plasma, then most of it will be dissolved in adipose tissue and cell membranes, and these things are not in the plasma. In this situation, the measured plasma drug concentration would be much lower than you would expect if the drug were present only in the plasma. The same is also true for highly protein bound drugs. Such drugs not only bind to plasma proteins, but also bind to proteins outside the plasma, which means that the measured plasma drug concentration is much lower than you would expect if the drug were only present in the plasma. I could go on and on with more examples, but the physiological volumes shown in Table 3.2 give an idea of the relationship of various pharmacokinetic volumes of drugs listed in the appendix to known body fluid compartment sizes. When combined with known physicochemical properties of drugs, this table also gives some insights into the reasons why pharmacokinetic volumes such as $V_c$ and $V_d$ are different to these physiological volumes. Here is also a short list of some physicochemical considerations."

- Fat-soluble drugs diffuse readily through phospholipid cell membranes into, and out of cells. This means they rapidly diffuse into erythrocytes, and diffuse rapidly through capillary endothelial cells into extravascular fluids and cells. Accordingly, such drugs have a reasonably rapid onset of action, as well as a $V_c$ and a $V_d$ very much larger than the plasma volume. Examples of such drugs are Thiopental and Propofol.
- Highly ionized, or fat-insoluble drugs cannot dissolve in phospholipid cell membranes, and because of this they cannot pass through cell membranes to enter into cells. This means they can only diffuse out of capillaries through transcapillary pores, as well as through the interstices between capillary endothelial cells, a fact slowing their passage into extravascular tissues. This explains why such drugs have a slower onset of action than fat-soluble drugs, and also explains why they have a $V_c$ and a $V_d$ not much larger than the extracellular fluid volume. Examples of such drugs are the highly ionized muscle relaxant drugs.

- Highly protein bound drugs have a $V_c$ and $V_d$ which is larger than the plasma volume, because they not only bind to plasma proteins, but also bind to proteins outside the plasma volume. Examples of such drugs are the opiates.

"This should make the relationship between pharmacokinetic volumes and physicochemical properties of drugs a little clearer. In the meantime, I do believe Bert would also like a cup of coffee. So it's back to the hell of the Crippen operating theater for you. I can't image he's finished yet. Give Hawley my regards, and thank him for his advice to leave the operating theater. I'm going to drink another cup of coffee."

Bob understood the lesson had come to an abrupt end. Feeling somewhat dazed with this information overload, he slowly stood up and shuffled back to the operating theater wondering why he always seemed to get this particular operating list.

# 4

# Paralyzed for hours

Today was different. Today Doctor Bob was going to administer anesthesia for a type of surgery he had never encountered before—a family donor kidney transplantation. A healthy man was going to donate one of his kidneys to his brother who had already undergone bilateral nephrectomy for renal failure caused by repeated, devastating pyelonephritis secondary to pyelolithiasis. One kidney of the healthy man would be removed, after which it would be transplanted into his anephric brother. Bob knew this was going to be a long day—true, a possibly an interesting and challenging day—but a long day nonetheless.

Bob had done his homework. He had studied the pharmacology of anesthetic drugs in relation to renal disease, so he was prepared for any questions Doctor Gerry might throw at him. After making his preparations for administering general anesthesia to the kidney donor, he made his way to find his mentor. Gerry was in his usual place in the coffee room, sitting, half asleep, one hand wrapped around a cup of strong black coffee, while hanging over a popular gossip magazine.

The transplant surgeon, Doctor Henry Bigelow entered the coffee room at the same time. Bigelow was an irascible man with a penchant for heavy-handed humor. He looked disapprovingly at Gerry, hissed softly, and remarked in an irritated tone dripping with sarcasm, "Ah, Gerry, I see you're absorbed in your professional literature. I almost don't dare interrupt such serious study, but instead of dreaming about gassing movie stars, why don't you move yourself into the operating theater and anesthetize the kidney donor."

"Oh it's you Henry, I was wondering when you would finally arrive. Gripping stuff in this magazine—good surgical articles too. Tell you what, I'll let you read this while Bob and I anesthetize the patient. You might even find a few good tips." Gerry drank the rest of his coffee, turned to Bob and said, "Good morning Bob. If you're ready, let's go."

The operating theater was cold. Bigelow always insisted on the air conditioning being adjusted to as low a temperature possible. Bob knew what Gerry was going to do once given the opportunity—he realized he was not only going to have a long day, but also a very cold day. Mr. Calculus, the healthy brother of the kidney patient lay on the operating table, and shortly afterwards was unconscious under general anesthesia. Bigelow scrubbed his hands during the induction, and walked into the operating theater just as Bob finished adjusting the ventilator settings.

During disinfection and draping of the patient for the operation, Gerry asked, "Tell me Bob, what is the difference in anesthetic technique between a donor nephrectomy performed on a brain dead patient with a beating heart, and a healthy living family donor."

Bob responded immediately—this was something he knew. "There is really very little difference. Both patients need muscle relaxants to prevent spinal cord mediated reflex muscle spasm, as well as opiates to diminish these same reflexes. The only real difference is that the brain dead donor is already unconscious, eternally unconscious, because he is dead. So you don't need to maintain unconsciousness in such patients." A pawky glint appeared in his eyes as he added in a cheerful voice, "But there is a big difference in the reversal of anesthesia. With the healthy family donor you wait until they regain consciousness and start breathing again before you disconnect the ventilator!"

Bigelow glared at Bob. "Hmmm..." was heard from Gerry, who now understood that Bob also had the same way as he of coping with the sometimes cruel realities of medical practice. "Quite right."

Shortly after the operation started, Gerry began to get restless. He walked around the operating table, inspected the suction pots, the drapes, and the floor around the feet of the surgeon. He peered in the wound, saw all was under control, sniffed loudly, tapped Bob on his shoulder and said, "I'm off to my room. Call me when it's ready." Bob sighed. The life of a resident was not easy.

The nephrectomy proceeded reasonably efficiently, and after about two and a half hours Bob brought the healthy donor into the recovery room. Shortly afterwards the anephric brother was wheeled into the operating theater. The brother of Mr. Calculus was quite different to his healthy sibling. He weighed about 70 kg, had a grey complexion and a sickly appearance. Bob inserted a drip into one of the few veins left over from the ravages of years of medical treatment and dialysis, and called Doctor Gerry.

Gerry arrived soon afterwards, studied the syringes of anesthetic drugs prepared for the anesthetic, and turned to Bob. "Hmmm... Atracurium... Now why don't you want to use Sugammadex to antagonize and mop up the muscle relaxant molecules if you're worried about muscle relaxants working too long? With Sugammadex you can completely antagonize Rocuronium or Vecuronium within minutes. Much better than Atracurium."

"Well Gerry, I've a number of questions about Sugammadex. It's got a molecular weight of about 2002 g/mole, binds irreversibly with the muscle relaxants such as Vecuronium and Rocuronium, which increases the molecular weight to something over 2600 g/mole (Appendix). Now I know that Sugammadex is mainly excreted unchanged in the urine (4), and because the molecular sieve size for the glomeruli is about 60,000 g/mole, I'm not worried about accumulation in people with normal renal function. But I don't know what happens when you administer it to anephric people, or people with severely reduced renal function. What happens to all those macromolecules then? Does the reticuloendothelial system mop them up, or what? Do these retained macromolecules have any adverse effects? These unknowns are my reasons for choosing Atracurium."

"Actually Bob, I'm also not too certain what the long term consequences are either. Sugammadex apparently doesn't undergo metabolic breakdown (4), and doesn't seem to cause any problems when administered to people with renal failure (5). Furthermore, it antagonizes non-depolarizing muscle relaxants such as Vecuronium and Rocuronium just as well in normal people as in those with renal failure (5). However, today we're not going to make it easy for ourselves by using Rocuronium and Sugammadex. Instead, we're going to exercise our minds, as well as employing such clinical acumen as we possess by using good old-fashioned Pancuronium as a muscle relaxant!"

"But, I've already drawn up an ampoule of Atracurium," protested Bob.

"Even so, we'll still use Pancuronium," was Gerry's resolute answer.

Bob remained silent, sensing that a learning moment was about to come. After induction and stabilization, he turned to Gerry and asked, "Isn't Pancuronium contraindicated in renal failure? After all, during the first 24 hours after administration of a dose of Pancuronium in normally healthy people, about 60% is excreted unchanged in the urine, while the rest is metabolized and excreted in bile and urine (1, 2). So the duration of action of

Pancuronium can be considerably prolonged in anuric renal failure patients, simply because it's elimination from the body and the resulting plasma elimination are much slower than normal. Atracurium is a better choice because it is not eliminated by metabolism in any organ—Atracurium molecules are unstable at body pH, breaking down spontaneously into inactive metabolites, which is why its elimination from the body, as well as its plasma elimination are not prolonged in renal failure patients."

"Well Bob, tell me how you think anesthesia was administered for renal transplantation before Atracurium and similar drugs became available in the middle 1980's?"

"A good question," was Bob's response. "I don't know. Tell me."

"Depending upon availability, as well as the preferences of the anesthesiologists, Tubocurare, Alcuronium, and Pancuronium were all used. And despite these drugs, the patients never remained paralyzed for hours after the operation unless they were myasthenic, or the anesthesiologist injected too much. The advantage of drugs such as Pancuronium, Vecuronium, and Rocuronium are that they cause a lot less histamine release and hypotension than do Atracurium or Mivacurium. Even so, I must admit these last two drugs are a better choice nowadays, simply because their elimination is independent of renal and hepatic function."

"Hey," interrupted Bigelow, "Can I begin with the operation? After all, this patient came for a kidney transplant, not a lesson on the advantages of one sort of deadly Indian arrow poison over the other."

"Okay, get on with it Henry before the anesthetic wears off. Now Bob, let's get on with our work and dispel this magical thinking you seem to have about the use of muscle relaxants in patients with renal failure. I don't want to know where you get these ideas, but once you hear how matters really are, you can go and spread the true facts. Now get your table of kinetic and dynamic parameters out, we're going to do a few calculations!"

Bob realized Gerry was in his unstoppable teaching mode. Gerry was going to teach him whether he wanted it or not. He sighed. Even so, he was interested in how Gerry was going to justify something he had read and heard was wrong.

Gerry began. "Get ready, we're going to perform some really complex calculations with mind-numbingly advanced mathematical techniques such as addition, subtraction, multiplication, and... steel yourself... division! Let's compare the durations of action of Pancuronium and Atracurium for Mr. Calculus."

"I almost can't wait," groaned Bob. "My floating-point synapses are already tingling with excitement."

- The weight of Mr. Calculus = 70 kg.
- Let's look at the situation after 60 minutes, a time far short of what is needed to complete the average kidney transplantation.

**Atracurium data (see Appendix)**
- Dose for most people would be about = 30 mg = 30/70 = 0.43 mg/kg.
- $t_{1/2\alpha} = 2$ min.
- $V_c = 0.07$ l/kg.
- $V_d = 0.32$ l/kg.
- $EC_{90}$ = concentration required for adequate surgical relaxation = 1.13 mg/1.
- Initial plasma concentration before any distribution or elimination have occurred = Dose/$V_c$ = 0.43/0.07 = 6.14 mg/1, which is a concentration far above that necessary for adequate surgical relaxation.

- Plasma concentration after distribution is complete (about 3 times $t_{1/2\alpha}$ = 3 x 2 = 6 min), and assuming no elimination has occurred = Dose/$V_d$ = 0.43/0.32 = 1.34 mg/1, which is a concentration still sufficient for adequate surgical relaxation.
- Now 60 minutes is a time equal to three times the $t_{1/2\beta}$ of Atracurium, which means that 87.25% of this dose of Atracurium will have been eliminated after 60 minutes.
- In other words, supplementary doses of Atracurium will be required before 60 minutes have elapsed.

**Pancuronium data (see Appendix)**
- Dose = most people would use a dose of 4 mg for an average adult = 4/70 = 0.06 mg/kg.
- $t_{1/2\alpha}$ = 10.7 min.
- $V_c$ = 0.12 l/kg.
- $V_d$ = 0.3 l/kg.
- $EC_{90}$ = concentration required for adequate surgical relaxation = 0.27 mg/1.
- Initial plasma concentration before any distribution or elimination have occurred = Dose/$V_c$ = 0.06/0.12 = 0.5 mg/1, which is a concentration double that required for adequate surgical relaxation.
- Plasma concentration after distribution is complete (about 3 times $t_{1/2\alpha}$ = 3 x 10.7 = 33 min.), and assuming no elimination has occurred = Dose/$V_d$ = 0.06/0.3 = 0.2 mg/1, which is a concentration insufficient to induce adequate surgical relaxation in this man.
- But after 60 minutes, some Pancuronium will have been eliminated by hepatic metabolism, even in anephric patients, so the concentration will actually drop even further below that required for surgical paralysis.

- In other words, supplementary doses of Pancuronium will be required before 60 minutes have elapsed.

"So," said Gerry, "there you are. You can use either drug in patients with renal failure. However, it is true you cannot use Pancuronium (or other non-depolarizing muscle relaxants for that matter), with as much freedom as Atracurium. Another interesting fact revealed by performing this type of equation for all non-depolarizing muscle relaxants, is that after times equal to three times their distribution half-lives, the plasma concentrations of many non-depolarizing muscle relaxant drugs resulting from normal clinical doses of these drugs will drop below the $EC_{90}$, the concentration at which a surgeon can perform a laparotomy without any difficulty due to reflex abdominal muscle spasm (Table 4.1)."

**Table 4.1**

| Drug | Clinical dose (mg/kg) | $t_{1/2\alpha}$ (min) | $V_d$ (l/kg) | $C_{plasma}$ at end of distribution = Dose/$V_d$ (mg/l) | $EC_{90}$ (mg/l) |
|---|---|---|---|---|---|
| Gallamine | 1 | 6.7 | 0.23 | 4.34 | 7.2 |
| Tubocurarine | 0.25 | 6.2 | 0.39 | 0.64 | 0.63 |
| Alcuronium | 0.3 | 13.8 | 0.4 | 0.75 | 0.66 |
| Pancuronium | 0.06 | 10.7 | 0.3 | 0.2 | 0.27 |
| Vecuronium | 0.08 | 7.5 | 0.4 | 0.084 | 0.15 |
| Rocuronium | 0.4 | 14.8 | 0.21 | 1.9 | 2 |
| Atracurium | 0.4 | 2 | 0.2 | 1.9 | 1.13 |
| Mivacurium | 0.15 | ? | 0.2 | 0.75 | 0.1 |

By the time Gerry was finished explaining all these things, about 45 minutes had passed since administration of the initial 4 mg of Pancuronium. "I do believe a moment of pharmaco- (or whatever you call it), decision making has arrived," came the irritated voice of Bigelow from the other side of the sterile drape hung between the anesthetic and the surgical parts of Mr. Calculus. (Some anesthesiologists jokingly refer to this sterile drape as the blood-brain barrier.) "I can't operate when the abdominal muscles are this tight. Do something," snarled Bigelow.

"This is a real cry for help Bob. So what are you going to do about it? According to me, you've got three choices: do nothing (which is hardly acceptable), give an extra dose of Pancuronium, or give a dose of Atracurium."

Bob had a moment of inspiration—he quickly looked over the blood-brain barrier into the wound, saw the operating field was neat and relatively free of blood, and also saw that Bigelow still had to place the transplant kidney. This would take about another hour. So without any further ado he injected one milligram of Pancuronium and gave some extra Sufentanil. "Just a moment Henry, and the Pancuronium will start working and you'll be able to proceed." Sounds of surgical contentment were heard soon afterwards: sounds of instructions to scrub nurses to pass and use instruments, the sounds of suction, as well as the intermittent sound of diathermy apparatus, all interspersed with the happy sounds of normal inconsequential surgical chatter.

"Really Bob—such decisiveness. Tell me why you gave Pancuronium instead of Atracurium."

Bob responded as decisively as he had acted. "I still think it would have been better to use Atracurium. Then we wouldn't even have to think whether it was safe to give another dose. But instead we used Pancuronium. I didn't administer a dose of Atracurium in this situation because I was worried about causing a dual block if I used these two relaxants together, so I administered a repeat dose of Pancuronium instead. I reasoned that some of the initial dose of Pancuronium was already certainly eliminated according to our discussion, and after another hour, even more will have been eliminated. So the extra dose of Pancuronium shouldn't give any problems. I calculate that we could even give a total dose of 6 mg Pancuronium to this man with reasonable impunity. After all, if you divide this dose by his weight of 70 kg, the dose per kilo will be $= 6/70 = 0.085$ mg/kg. Such a dose will result in a plasma Pancuronium concentration after full distribution without any elimination $= Dose/V_d = 0.085/0.3 = 0.27$ mg/l. True, this Pancuronium concentration is equal to the $EC_{90}$ for muscle relaxation, but even though Pancuronium elimination is considerably slowed by renal failure, after $45 + 60 = 105$ minutes operating time, a reasonable proportion will have been metabolized by the liver, because hepatic elimination is also a significant mode of elimination for Pancuronium, even in patients with renal failure."

"Your reasoning with Pancuronium is correct. You also estimated the necessary time to finish the operation by checking on the actual surgical situation yourself. I like that Bob. It indicates you don't trust the sometimes wildly optimistic opinions of surgeons. Well done. As regards the use of other muscle relaxants in persons with compromised renal function, the same principles apply as with Pancuronium. You can usually administer the initial dose with impunity. However, extra doses should always be administered with caution and some knowledge of how these drugs are eliminated from the body. In general, all drugs which are also eliminated via the liver, and which do not have an excessively long plasma elimination half-life can be used in patients with compromised renal function."

"Now for something else..." Gerry looked grim. His expression darkened as he said, "But there was another part of your answer which did not please me one little bit. Where, oh where did you ever hear this superstitious drivel about dual block being due to using two different muscle relaxants?"

Bob began to answer, but was cut short by Gerry. "I don't really want to know Bob. I'm even surprised you weren't struck by bolts of lightning sent down by the collective pantheon of the ever-observant anesthetic gods and saints for daring to mouth such utter twaddle! Really... Unbelievable! Let's look at the situation. Pancuronium and Atracurium are both neuromuscular blocking agents competing with Acetylcholine (Ach) for place on the Ach-receptors. If you compare the molecular weights and the dosages of both drugs you can immediately see that you need more molecules of Atracurium for a given degree of muscle relaxation than you need molecules of Pancuronium. But despite this evident difference in Ach-receptor affinity, they both act at the same place on the same receptors, and have the same actions. So you can actually use them interchangeably without any real problem. Just use the normal dosages of each."

Gerry continued, "Dual block is something quite different. Dual block occurs when you administer Succinylcholine too rapidly, or in too high a dose. This causes the normal depolarizing block due to Succinylcholine to change into a neuromuscular block with the same properties as a competitive neuromuscular blockade, such as is caused by all competitive neuromuscular blockers. You can even antagonize this dual block (otherwise known as a phase-2 block), with Neostigmine and Atropine (3). This is the definition of dual block. A dual block does not occur when you administer a nondepolarizing muscle relaxant shortly after Succinylcholine administration. The only thing that occurs then is that the two different types of relaxant antagonize each other, but that is also not a dual block, just antagonism. After all, as regards this latter antagonism, the Succinylcholine molecule is no more than two Acetylcholine molecules attached end-to-end to each other—a chemical combination resulting in a long acting form of Acetylcholine causing prolonged depolarization—the familiar depolarizing neuromuscular blockade of Succinylcholine."

"Now we come to more serious matters. I see the operation isn't finished yet, so I'm off to do other things. Call me when it's ready."

Bob knew this meant that Gerry was off for more coffee. He dreamed one day he too would be able to depart from the operating theater so easily leaving the resident behind—a situation that seemed to him like paradise at that moment. It was cold in the operating theater. So Bob threw a warm flannel sheet over his shoulders, sat down next to the anesthetic machine, started filling in the anesthetic chart, and listened to the sounds of surgical conversation. The subject matter shifted from matters related to the operation, to restaurants, and finally to holidays—especially about holidays in warmer climates. Bob groaned, "Ohhhh, the suffering, the suffering..."

# 5

## Blood loss, drug loss

Gerry sat in his room, musing in front of a thick questionnaire. He had finished all his correspondence. Now he was steel-
ing himself to fill in this example of yet another in a seemingly
interminable series of questionnaires that the middle management
types of Saint Elders Hospital took a perverse, even satanic delight in sending to medical specialists—possibly with the intention
of driving them insane with exasperation. He sighed. Unfortunately his presence in the operating theater was not needed, because
his resident, Bob, was doing well, learning fast and very adept
with most aspects of anesthesia. In fact Gerry did not need to
actively supervise him at all for most standard operations. But
now he had delayed filling in the questionnaire long enough. He
picked up his pen to begin, but was thankfully interrupted by Bob
on the intercom."

"Could you come to the operating theater Gerry, I'd like your
opinion on some problems here."

"Anything to delay the inevitable," thought Gerry as he
walked to the operating theater. Once inside he saw a full suction
pot containing at least two liters of blood. There was a liberal
amount of blood on the drapes around the abdominal wound,

which looked messy with edematous peritoneum, and blood oozing slowly from wound surfaces. Even so, it was evident from the height attained by a trail of blood on the mask and cap of the surgeon, Doctor Theo Billroth, that hypotension was definitely not a problem. The anesthetic chart revealed a blood loss of three liters, as well as the information that large doses of muscle relaxant and opiate had been administered.

Gerry liked Billroth, respected his skill as a surgeon, as well as the fact he always did his best for his patients. He began, "How's it going Theo? It looks like you've managed to find another one of those desperately awful gastrointestinal patients again. I always wonder where you manage to find them—or do they find you?"

"Hello Gerry. Yes, as usual the abdomen is full of adhesions, and the intestines are the usual inflamed rubbish that bleed the moment you touch them, but I've mobilized everything I need to mobilize, and the tissue planes are only oozing slightly now. All I need do now is perform the resection and make a stoma. So everything's under control. As to where these patients come from—I haven't the slightest idea. All I know is that I seem to get an unending stream of them from my wretched colleagues. Apparently they think I really enjoy operating on patients like these. Sometimes I wonder why I ever specialized in gastrointestinal surgery."

"Well Theo, I guess you've got a lot of bad karma to work away, otherwise you would have been an anesthesiologist." He turned to Bob, and asked, "So Bob, tell me what seems to be the problem."

"This patient is a Mr. Mikulicz who is undergoing an extensive ileocecal resection for therapy resistant Crohn's disease. There are two problems here: blood loss, and the fact that I have to give what I consider to be enormous doses of opiates and muscle relaxant drugs. I understand the cause of the blood loss—the colon, distal small intestine, and the surrounding tissues are inflamed due to Crohn's disease, so it is quite understandable that local hemostasis isn't optimal. I've replaced all the fluid and blood losses, so this is no real problem. But I can't understand why this man needs such high doses of anesthetic drugs. I'm almost afraid to administer any more muscle relaxant or opiate for fear I might have to ventilate him postoperatively."

"You're quite correct about the cause of the blood loss, but as you say, there's not much the surgeon or we can do about it. Let's talk about the unexpected, inordinately high doses of anesthetic drugs. To begin with, I wouldn't worry too much about high doses of anesthetic drugs. Our work is to administer anesthesia for the operation. If the patient needs high doses of anesthetic drugs, then the patient should receive these high doses, and we must adjust our management accordingly. Even so, it is interesting to know why the patient needs such high doses. So tell me Bob, why do you think Mr. Mikulicz requires such high doses of anesthetic drugs?"

Bob sensed a learning moment was about to begin. He was going to have to be very careful with what he now said. Gerry was merciless with all things he considered superstition, and equally merciless with all those who could not provide good arguments for their answers. Billroth also understood what was happening. He recognized the signs, he sighed, he knew Gerry was unstoppable once started with a lesson, and continued with his work in stoic silence. The scrub and circulating nurses also came to the dreadful realization that an anesthetic learning moment was about to begin. They knew from experience that this was the end of chatter for a while. Just at that moment the relief for the circulating nurse walked into the theater, enabling her to make a hasty and joyous escape to the coffee room. No such escape was possible for the scrub nurse. She looked unhappy, whimpered softly behind her mask, and continued passing instruments to Billroth in despondent silence.

"Well Bob?" were the expectant words of Gerry. "I'm waiting. This is not a difficult question."

"I was just thinking about how to formulate my answer a bit better," was Bob's reaction. "I had a similar, but not such extreme situation a few weeks ago when I was working with Doctor Trottel (another anesthesiologist in Saint Elders Hospital). We were also using Sufentanil and Rocuronium. According to him, so much Sufentanil and Rocuronium were lost in the surgical bleeding, that the plasma concentrations of these drugs decreased to such low levels that frequent top-up doses of these drugs were needed to maintain adequate muscle relaxation and analgesia."

Gerry demonstratively rolled his eyes upwards as if beseeching the heavens for enough strength to continue. He evidently found this strength, for he rapidly turned to Bob with the severe expression of an inquisitor about to root out some particularly nasty, perverse, and filthy heresy. The realization began to dawn upon Bob that this was perhaps not quite the answer Gerry wanted to hear, a realization born out by the stern and censorious tone of Gerry's response to his answer. "Are you telling me that you accepted this explanation without any criticism, or requests for proof?"

"Er... it seems a reasonable and logical answer," responded Bob, although he now began to suspect that this might not be the case.

"Ohhhhh... That Trottel... I see we have some work ahead of us. To begin with, how long has the present operation lasted, and how much blood has been lost? What are the normal blood, plasma, and extracellular fluid volumes in the human body? Furthermore, what are the volumes of distribution as well as the distribution half-lives of Rocuronium and of Sufentanil? Let's put this all in a list starting with the pharmacokinetic parameters."

**Sufentanil data (see Appendix)**
- $t_{1/2\alpha}$ = 1.4 minutes.
- $V_c$ = 0.16l/kg.
- $V_d$ = 2.9 l/kg.

**Rocuronium data (see Appendix)**
- $t_{1/2\alpha}$ = 14.8 minutes.
- $V_c$ = 0.038 l/kg.
- $V_d$ = 0.21 l/kg.

**Timing and human fluid compartment volumes**
- Blood volume in a normal male = 0.07 l/kg.
- Plasma volume = 0.04 l/kg.
- Extracellular fluid volume = 0.2 l/kg.
- Duration of operation at the moment of Gerry's arrival = 2 hours.
- Blood loss at the moment of Gerry's arrival = 3 liters.
- Blood loss occurred during the 1.5 hours before Gerry's arrival.

"Now Bob are you beginning to see where we're going."

"I believe so. I see that the volumes of distribution of both drugs are much larger than even the blood volume of the patient, all of which makes it very unlikely that the total amounts of these drugs within the body would be significantly affected by a blood loss of three liters."

"Quite right. But you've missed a few refinements based upon the actual clinical situation as well as the pharmacokinetics of the drugs used."

"You mean there's more?"

"Indeed. The blood loss occurred gradually over one and a half hours—which is 90 minutes—a time far longer than the duration of distribution for either Sufentanil or Rocuronium. So these drugs were totally distributed throughout their volumes of distribution at the time of blood loss. The volumes of distribution of anesthetic drugs are almost totally extravascular, which means that after distribution throughout their volumes of distribution, only a very small proportion of the doses of anesthetic drugs are actually present in blood. This is the reason why the amounts of anesthetic drugs lost in peroperative bleeding are minimal! Accordingly, loss of anesthetic drugs in peroperative bleeding is not the reason why this patient needs high doses of Sufentanil and Rocuronium."

"I understand all that," responded Bob. "It's quite evident from what you say that the majority of the administered doses of anesthetic drugs are present in their volumes of distribution in extravascular tissues, which is why minimal amounts of anesthetic drugs are lost due to surgical bleeding. But we replace surgical blood losses with volume expanding fluids and blood, and these fluids contain no anesthetic drugs. This means that losses of the minimal amounts of drugs present in blood due to surgical bleeding, together with dilution of the remaining amounts of these drugs with volume replacing fluids will quite dramatically reduce the plasma concentrations of anesthetic drugs in the circulation. According to me, this is the reason why this patient needs higher doses of anesthetic drugs than normal." And Bob looked at Gerry with a smug expression that said, "This is the true explanation. Now I understand..."

Gerry sighed—the sigh of a parent patiently correcting an erring child, "Oh, oh, oh, Bob. Diffusion of drugs into extravascular tissues is not one-way traffic. Drugs diffuse out of extravascular tissues back into the circulation when the plasma concentrations of these drugs are lower than their concentrations in extravascular tissues. Look at the molecular weights of all anesthetic drugs, and you see they all have molecular weights lower than 10,000 grams/mole (Appendix), which means they can all diffuse rapidly through capillary endothelium. Drug losses due to surgical bleeding, together with dilution due to volume replacing fluids does indeed cause the plasma concentrations of anesthetic drugs to decline, but rapid diffusion of these same drugs back into the circulation from the larger stores of these drugs present in extravascular tissues sustains the concentrations of these drugs at levels predicted by the normal pharmacokinetic equations."

"I guess you're right," said Bob. "I hadn't thought of it in that way before."

"There is however a rather dramatic way blood loss can significantly affect the total amount of anesthetic drugs in the body," continued Gerry. "If the patient rapidly loses one to three liters of blood at the same time as these drugs are administered intravenously, then anesthetic drug losses will be pharmacologically significant. But this is a very unlikely situation in clinical practice. What do think about all this Bob?"

Bob looked excitedly at his table of pharmacokinetic parameters (Appendix). "When you look at this table, you can see that the same reasoning applies to just about all anesthetic drugs. It's obvious when you look at it in the way you just explained it!"

"I'm so glad I was able to give you such a thrilling aha-experience Bob. But now tell me with your newly won knowledge just why this patient, as well as others in similar situations require higher doses of anesthetic drugs than normally healthy people."

"If blood loss is not the reason, then I can't imagine a pharmacokinetic reason. Do people with chronic intestinal inflammation have a high cardiac output causing faster distribution and elimination?"

**Table 5.1**

| Opiate | % protein bound (mainly to AAG) |
| --- | --- |
| Morphine | 35% |
| Meperidine | 50% |
| Methadone | 80% |
| Alfentanil | 92% |
| Fentanyl | 85% (mainly to albumin and lipoproteins) |
| Sufentanil | 93% |
| Remifentanil | 70% |

**Table 5.2**

| Muscle relaxant | % protein bound (muscle relaxnts mainly bind to albumin and much less to AAG) |
| --- | --- |
| Tubocurarine | 50% |
| Pancuronium | 10% |
| Vecuronium | 69% |
| Rocuronium | 45% |
| Atracurium | 37% |
| Mivacurium | 30% |

"Not always," replied Gerry, "an elevated cardiac output certainly does speed up distribution and may speed up elimination, but that is not the only reason in this case. However you did mention the basic reason—the altered physiology of people with chronic inflammatory diseases. The physiology of people with chronic and acute inflammation due to disease, infection, or severe injury is different to healthy people in that they make all manner of inflammation associated plasma proteins, among which is one called alpha-1-acid glycoprotein (AAG). This protein is present in the blood of normal healthy people too, but is present in much higher concentrations in the blood of people with acute and chronic inflammatory diseases, as well as in those suffering from severe injuries. Many anesthetic drugs bind to AAG to a greater or lesser degree, although opiates in particular bind to AAG. So what do you think is the anesthetic consequence of the increased plasma AAG concentration in the blood of people with chronic inflammatory disease? I'll make it easy for you by showing you a table of the percentage protein binding of some opiates and muscle relaxants (Tables 5.1 and 5.2)."

Bob looked at these tables and began to feel inspired. "All anesthetic drugs act on tissues outside the blood vessels. Only free drug, unbound to plasma proteins can diffuse out of the capillaries into the extravascular tissues to exert an effect. Plasma AAG concentrations are increased in people with chronic and acute inflammatory disorders, as well as in those with severe injuries. With exception of Fentanyl which mainly binds to plasma albumin and plasma lipoproteins, most opiates bind mainly to AAG, while muscle relaxants bind to AAG to a much lesser extent. Higher concentrations of plasma AAG means there is a higher proportion of plasma protein-bound drug unavailable for causing a drug effect, so perhaps the effects of muscle relaxants, but certainly the effects of many opiates are reduced in people with chronic and acute inflammatory disorders, as well as in those with severe injuries. Sufentanil and Rocuronium bind mainly to plasma AAG, and because of this, lower proportions of the doses of these drugs are available for diffusion into extravascular tissues where they act. This explains why this patient needs so much Sufentanil and Rocuronium."

"Quite right Bob. You're getting reasonably good at this type of reasoning. I'm beginning to believe you may even begin to understand the basics of practical pharmacokinetics and pharmacodynamics by the end of this year. There is one more thing with this patient. I do believe he also has an elevated cardiac output. Elevated cardiac output will certainly speed up distribution of nearly all intravenously administered drugs, so reducing their distribution half lives, and this would also partly account for the fact that the Sufentanil and Rocuronium you administered seem to act shorter than normal."

"Got him! It's pay-back time!" thought Bob as he asked, "How can you say his cardiac output is elevated when we haven't even measured it? You tell me to only rely on measurements, but here we haven't a single shred of evidence for an elevated cardiac output."

"Oh yes we do. We have a capnograph, and that gives us two indirect measures of cardiac output. Firstly there is the indirect indication of cardiac output we can derive from the fact that Mr. Mikulicz is afebrile, is being ventilated at a rate of 16 breaths per minute with a tidal volume of about 10 ml/kg, yet his end-tidal $CO_2$ ($ETCO_2$) concentration is 6%. The fact that his respiratory minute volume is so high, while his $ETCO_2$ is still 6%, means he is producing a lot of $CO_2$ and removing it from his tissues at a higher than normal rate. $CO_2$ is transported to the lungs in blood, and the rate at which is transported to the lungs is determined by the cardiac output. The higher the cardiac output, the higher the rate of $CO_2$ transport to the lungs. So here we have indirect evidence that the cardiac output of this man is elevated."

"Then we come to the second and more direct measure of the cardiac output, which is the angle, or slope of the plateau of the capnogram. This is not a new method—it is a method of measuring cardiac output used by physiologists since the 1940's. The plateau phase of the capnogram occurs during expiration when

$CO_2$ from the alveoli enters the expired air. $CO_2$ from the better-ventilated alveoli determines the initial height of the plateau. As expiration progresses, $CO_2$ enters the expired air from the less well ventilated alveoli, and so the plateau is not entirely horizontal, but slopes upwards tending to equal the pulmonary capillary $CO_2$. When there are large differences between alveolar perfusion and speeds of alveolar emptying—as occurs in the inhomogeneous alveolar population of the lungs of people with chronic obstructive pulmonary diseases—the slope of the plateau can be quite pronounced. Furthermore, the flow of blood through the lungs continues during expiration, which means that $CO_2$ in blood flowing through the lungs also continually diffuses into the lungs during expiration. $CO_2$ diffuses into the lungs at a constant rate determined by the cardiac output pumping blood through the lungs. But this $CO_2$ diffuses into the lungs at a time when lung volume is contracting during expiration. This is another reason why the $CO_2$ concentration continually increases in exhaled air during the plateau phase, tending to equal the pulmonary capillary $CO_2$ concentration, but never exceeding it. Here is a drawing of the situation. The higher the cardiac output, the faster the rate of increase of the $CO_2$ concentration, or slope of the plateau as expressed by the Greek letter sigma ($\sigma$), and in people with healthy lungs, cardiac output is directly related to the slope of the capnogram during the plateau phase. Mr. Mikulicz does not have chronic obstructive pulmonary disease, which means he has a relatively homogeneous alveolar population in his lungs, but he does have a high slope in the plateau phase of his capnogram, indicating to me he has a high cardiac output."

"Wonderful! Amazing!" called the agitated voice of Billroth from the other side of the sterile drape. "But in case you hadn't noticed, the patient is moving. Hold him still! I only need to put in one or two more staples."

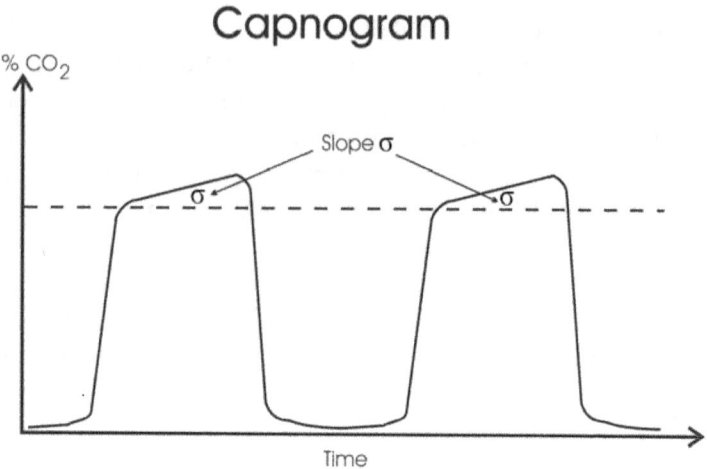

Figure 5.1: A typical capnogram curve of a person with normal lung function.

Just as the last staple was clicked into the skin wound, Mr. Mikulicz began coughing, attempted to remove his endotracheal tube, while at the same time he attempted to break his bones by trying to roll off the operating table onto the hard concrete floor. He opened his eyes. He was awake, confused, and struggling wildly. All members of the anesthetic and surgical teams hurled themselves in unison upon his body to prevent him from rolling onto the floor. After a few minutes of wild struggle, Mr. Mikulicz calmed down and began to understand where he was.

"See Bob," said Gerry, "just as I said, a high cardiac output, and very probably also a high AAG concentration. That's why he needed so much, and that's why he woke up so rapidly. Let's put this man in bed, so that you and the nurse can bring him to the recovery room. Order the next patient, and call me when you're ready to start the induction."

With these last words Gerry departed to lave his parched throat with warm black coffee. Teaching certainly was exhausting and thirsty work. While walking to the coffee room, he sighed as he mentally paraphrased a very appropriate verse in the book of Ecclesiastes.

*And further, by these, my son, be admonished: of making many books there is no end, and much teaching is a weariness of the flesh. (1)*

So it was that Bob learnt the true facts about how blood loss and chronic disease can affect the pharmacokinetic and pharmacodynamic properties of anesthetic drugs.

# 6

## Corpulentia maxima

The perspiring bulk of Mr. A. Dipose was wheeled into the smallest operating theater at Saint Elders Hospital. His flabby 160 kilograms was a monument to many years avid spaghetti eating with rich sauces, potato crisps, snacks in between meals, nightly feasts, and many liters of calorie-rich vitamin-free drinks each day. Even so, his body was but a pale shadow of its once magnificent 220 kilograms, because Mr. A. Dipose had to lose a lot of weight before being accepted for a laparoscopic gastric banding procedure. He was motivated to lose weight and undergo this procedure after his body gave several subtle signs of imminent mortality secondary to obesity; one year before he had spent a month being ventilated in the intensive care for respiratory failure secondary to a Candida albicans sepsis and pneumonia, during which he was also found to have type-2 Diabetes mellitus, as well as suffering a mild myocardial infarction, and a deep venous thrombosis resulting in a pulmonary embolus.

Bob sighed at the thought of the anesthetic challenges presented by this patient, as well as the space-occupying and olfactory presences in the same small operating theater of Mr. A. Dipose together with the surgeon, Doctor Sam Pickwick. Sam Pickwick was also a cheerful junk-food fanatic, whose favorite diet consisted of large quantities of potato chips accompanied by hamburgers, and the quaffing of liberal amounts of calorie-rich Irish beer. This diet meant he was somewhat portly to say the least. And unfortunately, just like Mr. A. Dipose, he also perspired a lot.

The operating table was a multifunctional European wonder with a maximum load capacity rated at no more than 180 kg; people in Western Europe seldom ever get this heavy. It squeaked and groaned slightly as a loudly puffing Mr. A. Dipose rolled, squirmed, and wobbled from his bed onto the operating table.

"You could have helped by lifting me," panted Dipose in a plaintive tone as he settled on the table with his flanks hanging over both sides.

A drip was inserted into one of the few veins visible on one of his podgy hands, the monitoring was attached, and then it was time to start the induction. As usual, just at that moment, Gerry walked into the operating theater wafting a smell of coffee in his path. His nose wrinkled in response to the sudden olfactory confrontation with the truly wondrous variety of volatile molecules emanating from the immense body surface of Mr. A. Dipose. He sniffed, "So Bob I see it's time to begin. You intubate, and I'll inject."

Gerry continued talking as he injected one drug after the other. "Mr. Dipose, I'll first inject a powerful painkiller. It will probably make you feel like you've had a few drinks too many. Now for the sleeping drug... but before you fall asleep, you may notice some pain in your hand and arm. Sleep tight, and pleasant dreams."

But Mr. A. Dipose was still awake after having received 30 mcg Sufentanil and 200 mg Propofol. So Gerry quickly grabbed another syringe of Propofol and rapidly injected another 150 mg. Shortly afterwards, Mr. A. Dipose fell asleep, a fact rewarded by the administration of a large dose of a non-depolarizing muscle relaxant. Bob picked up the laryngoscope and inserted it into the mouth and throat of Mr. A. Dipose, upon which Mr. A. Dipose began waving his arms and legs. Gerry rapidly emptied the last 50 mg Propofol, as well as another 20 mcg Sufentanil into the patient. Finally, Mr. A. Dipose remained still during intubation and was connected to the ventilator. The surgical team was given the sign they could begin.

"Hey Sam, the operating table is loaded to almost maximum capacity, so if I was you I wouldn't lean too hard on the patient, unless you want your feet to be flatter than they already are," said Gerry.

"You're telling me this after all those liters of fluids and anesthetic drugs you just used. You lot just reduced the margin between the load capacity of the table and the weight of this patient. It's almost impossible for me to do anything. Just don't try drowning this man with excessive amounts of intravenous fluids, otherwise the whole lot will collapse," grumbled a good humored Pickwick as he began smearing iodine over the vastness of Mr. A. Dipose's bare abdomen.

Gerry and Bob moved the arms of Mr. A. Dipose into maximum abduction to give Pickwick more space to work. Bob quickly threw a warm flannel sheet over the upper chest, arms, and especially the axillae after seeing one of the scrub nurses suddenly gag, turn pale, and reel back while squeezing her nose after accidental exposure to the fragrance emanating from these dank and hairy pits. Soon Mr. A. Dipose was draped, and Pickwick began the operation. The sounds of clinking instruments, of suction, and of diathermy together with the smell of burning fat, followed by instructions to adjust the white balance and gas pressures, soon changed into the contented clucking of trivial surgical chatter. All was well on the other side of the sterile drape separating surgical and anesthetic worlds. On the anesthetic side—the patient was stable. It was time for a moment of anesthetic reflection and serious thought. Gerry turned to Bob with a by now well-known glint in his eyes. Bob knew this look—a learning moment was about to begin. The nurses also perceived this same glint—women are acutely perceptive of such social cues. The circulating nurse scurried off to join the surgical conversation, while Sister Patricia the anesthetic nurse suddenly discovered she needed to check the opiate cupboard in the main storeroom.

"Tell me Bob, what did you observe with this patient, and what can you tell me about reasons for the large total dose of Propofol we needed for induction of hypnosis?" began Gerry.

"Er..." began Bob, as his mind began to race over what he had seen, and what he expected Gerry might want to hear.

"Ur was the capital of the Chaldeans in ancient Mesopotamia," interrupted Gerry impatiently. "It was also the city in which Abraham, the founder of the Israelite nation was born more than 4000 years ago (1). But I don't want to hear what you know about Biblical history, I want to hear something about this patient."

Wheezing, snuffling, sniffling sounds, not unlike those made by an asthmatic dog with a harelip, were heard coming from Pickwick. "Good one Gerry," he snorted. Pickwick laughed at just about every joke, even the most appallingly weak ones. Gerry looked in the direction of Pickwick, rolled his eyes, groaned softly, and turned towards Bob with an inquiring look in his eyes.

Bob began hesitantly. "The induction dose of Propofol is somewhere between 2 to 3 mg/kg body weight. Okay, Mr. A. Dipose was anxious with a high cardiac output, so we can assume the higher dose requirement of 3 mg/kg was needed. His body weight is 160 kg, which means an induction dose = 160 x 3 = 480 mg. So an induction dose of 400 mg is not altogether unexpected, when you consider he also received a lot of Sufentanil prior to induction that would have reinforced the hypnotic action of the Propofol which you also injected at a very fast rate."

"Oh dear Bob, just as I was starting to think you might be learning a physiological approach, you come with a smidgen of physiology to make me happy, and for the rest you make do with cookbook medicine, otherwise known as package insert medicine. Are you trying to tell me that you think the amount of fat and other tissue making up the somewhat unsightly body of Mr. A. Dipose actually influenced the induction dose we used?"

"Yes, I do," responded Bob, "otherwise the initial 200 mg Propofol you gave him would have been sufficient to induce hypnosis in the usual arm-brain circulation time. Propofol is very fat-soluble with a $V_d = 4.7$ l/kg, so it is very reasonable to believe that Propofol distributes so rapidly in the body of an obese person that a higher induction dose is needed than for a person with a normal body composition. That's the explanation Dr. Trottel gave me last week when I worked with him on an almost identical patient. I must admit, it sounds like a very reasonable and logical explanation."

"Hmmm..." was Gerry's unexpectedly mild reaction to these words. "Well Bob, think back to what I told you about induction doses when we discussed them during the operation on the unfortunate Mrs. Elmore (see Chapter 3). So let's apply these same physiological and anatomical insights here too. When the Propofol was injected into Mr. A. Dipose, it first passed through his arm veins into his superior vena cava. Is there any fat along these blood vessels where this very fat-soluble Propofol can be rapidly absorbed?"

"Er... No," replied Bob.

"Okay, the Propofol then passes through the right atrium and right ventricle. Any fat there?"

"No..." Bob began to look unsure, wondering what Gerry was going to say next.

"The Propofol then passes through the pulmonary blood vessels to enter the left atrium and left ventricle. So tell me Bob, is there any fat in these structures where this extremely fat-soluble Propofol can be absorbed?"

Bob looked even more uncertain as he cautiously replied, "No…"

"Now this Propofol passes through the aorta, enters the carotid and vertebral arteries before finally passing into the brain capillaries. Is there any fat where this extremely fat-soluble Propofol can be absorbed before it enters these brain capillaries where it diffuses into brain tissues to induce consciousness in one arm-brain circulation time?"

Bob looked somewhat nonplussed as he answered, "No fat at all Gerry. It's quite obvious that fat absorption plays no role in determining the induction dose of Propofol. Dr. Trottel had it wrong. But this simple anatomical reality still leaves the question unanswered of why obese people need a higher induction dose of induction agents than people with a normal body composition. How would you explain this observation? And why does everyone express intravenous anesthetic induction doses in terms of body weight?"

"Well Bob, the total dose of an intravenous anesthetic induction agent needed to induce hypnosis actually does not correlate well with body weight at all. In fact, the only reason for expressing dosages of intravenous induction agents in terms of body weight is that it is a convenient way of saying that larger people often need larger induction doses of these drugs. Intravenous anesthetic induction dosages actually correlate better with lean body mass, cardiac output, central blood volume, and pulmonary blood volume better than with total body weight (2). So let's make a list of what we know, and use physiology to explain the induction dose of Propofol we administered to Mr. A. Dipose."

- Body weight of Mr. A. Dipose = 160 kg.
- Total induction dose of Propofol = 400 mg.

- Propofol is a very fat-soluble drug. This means it also diffuses into erythrocytes. Accordingly, we can make the very reasonable assumption that whole blood, and plasma Propofol concentrations are equal.
- A man with a body weight of about 80 kg would have a resting cardiac output of about 6 l/min. But Mr. A. Dipose weighs 160 kg, which is 80 kg more than our example man with a body weight of 80 kg. The extra weight of Mr. A. Dipose is nearly all adipose tissue. But even adipose tissue needs blood, although not as much blood as muscle, liver, kidney, or nervous tissues require. So his resting cardiac output would be about 8 l/min. Add a bit more for anxiety, and his resting cardiac output at the time of induction was perhaps about 9 l/min.
- Our 400 mg of Propofol was injected over a total time of 20 seconds, which meant it mixed with a volume of venous blood returning to the heart = 9 x 20/60 = 3 liters.
- Heart volume is normal in obese persons. So the combined volume of his right and left hearts is about 240 ml = 0.24 liter.
- Pulmonary blood volume is about 500 ml in normal adults, but is increased by as much as 50% in obese persons (3). Let's assume a pulmonary blood volume in Mr. A. Dipose of about 750 ml = 0.75 liter.
- This means the induction dose mixed with a total volume of blood = 3 + 0.24 + 0.75 = 3.99 liters.
- So after an induction dose of 400 mg Propofol administered over 20 seconds, the initial plasma concentration of Propofol in blood pumped by the heart of Mr. A. Dipose into his aorta from where it entered his coronary and systemic arteries = 400/3.99 = 100.25 mg/l. This was the ini-

tial Propofol concentration in the arterial blood going into the brain of Mr. A. Dipose.

- This initial concentration is rather less than that achieved with a 200 mg dose of Propofol in a person with a normal body build as we worked out in Chapter 2, but still much higher than the hypnotic concentration of Propofol (Table 2.1). This lower peak concentration also partly explains why he took somewhat longer to fall asleep than a person with a normal body weight.

"Very well," responded Bob, "but what you've done here is to substitute cookbook dosages with a sort of physiological fantasy. Okay, I agree some changes in cardiovascular physiology do occur in obese people, but are they really of such a magnitude? As regards the increased cardiac output—I also believe the cardiac output is increased in obesity, but how? After all, heart size, pulse rate and blood pressure are all reasonably normal in most obese people."

"These physiological changes due to obesity certainly do occur, and they are of these magnitudes. Let's have a look at what happens in obesity. When the left and right ventricles contract in normal people, they don't empty completely. The fraction of the end-diastolic volume pumped out of each ventricle of the heart is called the ejection fraction for that ventricle. Right and left ventricles are somewhat different. In people with a normal body weight, the right ventricular ejection fraction is about 0.5, which means that 50% of the end-diastolic volume is pumped out of the right ventricle per heartbeat, while the left ventricular ejection fraction is about 0.7, which means that 70% of the end-diastolic volume is pumped out of the left ventricle per heartbeat. Pulse rate and heart size are normal in obese people. So there is really only one way obese people can increase their cardiac outputs—some mechanism causes the ejection fractions of both ventricles to increase, increasing the stroke volume per heartbeat, as a result of which cardiac output is increased in obese people without significantly increasing heart size or pulse rate (4,5,6). Now Bob, what is a consequence of increased cardiac output on anesthetic drug action?"

Bob answered promptly, "This is something I've learned from our previous discussions. Increased cardiac output has two effects on drug pharmacokinetics: initial peak arterial plasma drug concentrations decrease with increasing cardiac output (7), and by increasing the speed of drug distribution throughout the body, increased cardiac output decreases the drug distribution half-life of many drugs (8,9). These effects increase the dosage requirements, and reduce the durations of anesthetic drug effects respectively. "

"Very good Bob, quite correct. Now here comes a difficult question. As you know, you can administer two basic types of general anesthesia to patients who receive muscle relaxants: you can administer a total intravenous anesthetic using intravenous hypnotic and opiate drugs, or you can administer an anesthetic vapor as hypnotic together with an opiate for analgesia. Which of these two is the better technique for obese patients?"

Bob thought about what he had read on this matter, thought about what he had heard from others, and reflected on his own experience. "A tricky question. Actually I can't give a single answer. The answer lies in the interaction between postoperative pain, and the well-known fact that obese people are more likely to develop postoperative hypoxia due to all causes than people with a normal body weight. But I would imagine that regardless of whether you used total intravenous anesthesia, or anesthesia supplemented with a vapor, that a technique using a higher opiate dosage relative to the concentration of vapor, or dosage of intravenous hypnotic, would be the better option. I believe this would be better, simply because obese people who have adequate postoperative analgesia after thoracic or upper abdominal surgery are less likely to develop postoperative hypoxia or respiratory failure."

"Well reasoned Bob. In fact the few published studies on this matter do seem to confirm this idea (10). Of course the best technique is to use a loco-regional technique for anesthesia in morbidly obese persons. So if general anesthesia is needed, then try and supplement the anesthetic with a loco-regional technique if possible. Now for something else—while you were busy answering my questions, the peripheral oxygen saturation ($S_pO_2$) of this man gradually decreased to 85%. Do something about it!"

Bob looked at the color of the patient to see if he was cyanotic, changed the position of the oxygen saturation meter sensor, as well as checking to see there were no disconnections, and that Mr. Dipose was indeed being ventilated and receiving oxygen. All these things convinced him that the measurement of an arterial oxygen saturation of 85% was true. He then checked the depth of the endotracheal tube, and whether the cuff was leaking. Finally he saw that the capnograph was reading an end-tidal $CO_2$ of 7%—the patient was being hypoventilated! So Bob gave a bit more head-up tilt (much to the delight of Pickwick), and increased the tidal volume as well as the rate of ventilation. A few minutes later the $S_pO_2$ was 95%. Bob was happy.

Pickwick was also happy, "Finally, almost reasonable anesthesia. Could you give me a bit more head-up tilt?"

"No," was Gerry's curt answer, "any more and the patient would be standing upright." A grumbling Pickwick proceeded with the operation as Gerry turned once more to Bob. "You first checked whether the patient was being ventilated and whether the measurement was correct. That's the way to do it. But tell me your reason for wanting to improve the saturation of this man. Were you afraid that a $S_pO_2 = 85\%$ would cause brain damage, cause loss of consciousness, or just alter his mental function? After all, you must have had a reason."

"Actually I don't know the $S_pO_2$ levels at which any of those things occur. All I know is that an $S_pO_2$ of 85% is abnormally low, and that hypoxia is not good for people." Bob began to warm to this chain of reasoning, and began to think he could finesse his way past this question. "So I improved his oxygenation, because regardless of what level all those things occur, desaturation is a sign something is not going well, and if something is not going well, the cause has to be investigated and corrected." As he finished this sentence he mentally added a, "So, there, eat them beans!"

"Hmmm... you're doing well today Bob. So I'll tell you the answer to the second part of my question. You're quite correct as regards the reason to improve the patient's oxygenation. But it is also useful to know what levels of hypoxia cause dysfunction, and what levels are actually harmful. Here it is in the form of a list derived from a wonderful book written by G.M. Woerlee called Mortal Minds (11)."

- Mild oxygen starvation occurs in the $S_pO_2$ range of 100-80%: Brain function is unaffected.
- Moderate oxygen starvation occurs in the $S_pO_2$ range of 80-60%: Brain malfunction occurs in this range, and the degree of brain malfunction worsens with increasingly severe hypoxia. This degree of hypoxia affects the functioning of the brain and the senses, removes sensations of pain or discomfort, causes people to feel calm, sometimes even joyful, as well as arousing feelings of serene unconcern or indifference. Supplementary motor cortex malfunction results in a lack of desire to move, so people usually do not move. A degree of primary motor cortex malfunction causes muscle weakness, so that when some

people do try to move, they discover that voluntary movement is difficult and requires intense effort. More severe degrees of moderate oxygen starvation may also induce life-review, or out-of-body experiences.

- Severe oxygen starvation occurs in the $S_pO_2$ range of 60-40%: This degree of oxygen starvation induces all the effects of moderate oxygen starvation, except that the degree of brain malfunction is more extreme. Supplementary and primary motor cortex malfunction are such that people do not even think of moving, and when a few people do try to move, they discover they are totally paralyzed. And because severely oxygen starved people do not move they appear unconscious, even though they are often still conscious.

- Extreme oxygen starvation occurs in the $S_pO_2$ range of 40-0%: This degree of hypoxia causes failure of all brain and brain-stem functions, causing loss of consciousness, abnormal, or actual cessation of breathing, and ultimately death.

"So Bob, as you see, this patient was not in any danger of developing hypoxic tissue damage in any of his organs. But the decreased saturation did signal that something was not right. In this case it was hypoventilation, although it could have been any one of a number of causes. Now I want to ask one last tricky question—at what $S_pO_2$ level can you detect cyanosis? You should know the answer, because the research on it was done about 60 years ago. Nothing new there at all."

Bob's mind was beginning to freeze up with all this new knowledge. He felt as if his head could take no more. "I really don't know," he said, "but I'll take a guess that a $S_pO_2$ of about 90% is when cyanosis becomes clinically visible to most people."

"Disappointing Bob... But I guess you must be tired by now. So I'll tell you the answer. Clinical investigation shows conclusively that cyanosis only becomes evident to most people at a $S_pO_2$ of 80% and lower, although some people can detect it at higher percentages (12). I think this is enough for one day. I also see that the gastric band has yet to be placed, which means this operation will last some time yet. So I'll be in the coffee room if you need me." With this last remark, Gerry strolled off to rinse his parched tonsils with a cup of delicious warm black coffee.

Left alone in the small dark operating theater with a bulky perspiring surgeon, and an even bulkier patient whose expansive body surface emanated all manner of wondrous, but odoriferous volatile substances, Bob began to get a distinctly self-pitying feeling that his existence was very similar to that of a mushroom—he was kept in the dark, and every now and then a load of manure was shoveled over him. He heaved a sad sigh as he started adding notes and measurements to the anesthetic chart.

# 7

# Feeding time

Doctor Bob checked the name, date of birth, allergies, and the planned operation against the information on the anesthetic chart as he wheeled Mrs. Suk Ling into the operating theater. Mrs. Suk Ling was a young, well-spoken and educated woman of Chinese origin who was to undergo an infundibulotomy under general anesthesia. She was also extremely nervous, and as Bob attached the usual anesthetic monitoring, she turned towards the ENT (ear, nose and throat) surgeon to ask him the big question burning on the tip of her tongue. "Oh Doctor Sluder, I breastfeed my three month old baby. Could you tell me how long I should stop breastfeeding after this operation."

Fred Sluder turned from the CT-scan of the sinuses containing the plentiful polyps he was soon to harvest. "Mrs. Suk Ling, I really don't know. I think you'd better ask Doctor Bob the anesthesiologist that question. He knows more about those things than I do. After all, he's specialized in anesthesia."

Mrs. Suk Ling was not especially pleased with this answer. It was a totally new concept for her, because she had always thought an anesthesiologist was some sort of nurse who just did what the surgeon asked. She looked towards Doctor Bob, and critically appraised his appearance. He was young and didn't look like a specialist. He looked like all the other blue-clad people in the operating theater. In fact, the appearance of Doctor Bob did not inspire her with any real confidence at all. Just as she was about to ask Bob the same question she asked Sluder, Doctor Gerry entered the operating theater wafting a strong smell of fresh coffee and garlic. Yet in spite of the strong smell of coffee and garlic, as well as the unruly graying hair protruding at all angles from under his cap, he was an imposing man whose presence oozed a sense of authority and calm. "This is a man who inspires confidence," she thought. "But who is he?"

Gerry greeted all in the operating theater, looked at the preoperative chart, and introduced himself to Mrs. Suk Ling. His certain and knowledgeable manner spoke volumes—she realized this was a man who could answer her question. "Oh doctor, I breastfeed my baby, and I've heard that anesthetic drugs stay in the body for several months. So is it safe to breastfeed my baby after general anesthesia, and if it's safe, how long after this operation must I wait before I can resume breastfeeding?"

"Good questions—questions that for some reason many people curiously find difficult to answer," replied Gerry. "But the answer is really quite simple. Anesthetic drugs are only administered during an operation, and awakening from anesthesia means that the concentrations of these anesthetic drugs in your brain, as well as in your blood are too low to keep you asleep. Now, nearly all drugs diffuse into, and out of mothers' milk via the bloodstream, and the flow of blood through breast tissue is quite high, which is why concentrations of anesthetic drugs in mothers' milk are about the same as in blood (1). All this means that anesthetic drug concentrations in mothers' milk are also low after awakening from anesthesia. Furthermore, anesthetic drugs almost totally disappear out of the blood after several hours, as do anesthetic drugs in mothers' milk."

Gerry continued, "So when you study the basic process of breastfeeding, you realize that a baby drinks milk with its mouth, but drinks no more than 40 to 200 milliliters per feed (2), which means that the total dose of anesthetic drugs ingested in milk during a single feed is very low. Mother's milk enters a baby's body through its mouth, and passes through the stomach into the intestines where it is digested, after which it is absorbed together with any drugs into the baby's body. Milk is digested slowly in the intestines, and all drugs, as well as all other substances entering the body through the intestines, first undergo substantial metabolism or breakdown in the liver before entering the circulation. When you think about all these things, you can readily appreciate that the total doses of anesthetic drugs entering the circulation of a baby as a result of breastfeeding are really very small. So the standard advice is simple—if you are capable of doing so, you can breastfeed your baby immediately after awakening from general anesthesia with modern anesthetic drugs. But if you are not up to it, use a breast pump, and resume breastfeeding later on when you feel fit enough. Does that answer your questions?"

Mrs. Suk Ling nodded uncertainly, "Yes, but anesthetic drugs are very dangerous, and I'm worried that even very small amounts may affect my baby."

"Mrs. Suk Ling, these minimal amounts of anesthetic drugs are also present in your body and cause you no harm, so even if by some pharmacological wonder your baby does experience some effects from the remaining miniscule amounts of anesthetic drugs in your milk, they won't harm him in any way either. And even if he is affected by these tiny amounts of anesthetic drugs, then at most he will be a little sleepy—an ideal situation for a mother recovering from an operation."

"Yes, I understand. A slightly sleepy baby after an operation sounds like heaven to me. But what about painkilling drugs? I may need to take painkillers for a while after my operation—will these affect my baby?"

"Painkilling drugs administered after operations are not a problem at all. Paracetamol is the painkiller used after almost all ENT operations, and maternal ingestion of this drug is safe for breastfeeding babies (1). As for other painkillers, it is best to avoid aspirin because of its association with Reye's syndrome, but maternal use of other painkillers such as the group of drugs called NSAID's (non-steroidal anti-inflammatory drugs), as well as Morphine, and other morphine-like drugs are also safe for breast-feeding babies (1). In fact, Meperidine is the only painkilling drug administered to nursing mothers after operations that is known to affect babies. Even so, this effect of Meperidine is only a slight perceived problem, because all it does is cause some changes in the behavior of nursing babies. But you won't be getting any of that old-fashioned rubbish here."

Mrs. Suk Ling heaved a grateful sigh of relief, "Yes. I understand, and I'm ready."

"Okay Bob, let's start." Upon these words Gerry injected the usual induction doses of Propofol, Alfentanil, and Rocuronium. Sluder got the sign to begin after the patient was intubated and stabilized. He asked whether he could insert the usual wads drenched in cocaine and epinephrine into her nose. "Go ahead, enjoy yourself, and do what you normally do. It won't have any effect on the ability of this woman to feed her baby." was Gerry's response.

Doctor Bob observed and heard all these things in silence, but now he cleared his throat, and began. "What you said all sounds very plausible. But is it true?"

"Of course it's true. I'm a doctor—would I lie to you? If you don't believe me, look at the plasma elimination half-lives of anesthetic drugs (Appendix). Look at the plasma concentrations needed for their effects. Look at the time scale in which we work, and you will see that all I told this woman is true. But there is another refinement I did not burden this woman with. About 4% of human milk (4 g/100 ml) is composed of lipids of all sorts, which is a lipid concentration very much higher than that in human plasma. Accordingly, concentrations of lipid-, or fat-soluble drugs are higher in mothers' milk than for the same drugs in plasma. This is also true for lipid-soluble anesthetic drugs. However, human brain is composed of about 10 to 12% of all manner of lipids, so the concentrations of anesthetic drugs in the maternal brain upon awakening are always much higher than in the plasma—and the mother is awake at this time. So it is evident that mothers' milk concentrations of anesthetic drugs are so low at the end of general anesthesia, that women can actually resume breastfeeding in the recovery room should they so desire."

"I believe you. But you also mentioned the period when people are administered drugs postoperatively. So what about the postoperative period, and especially what about Meperidine?"

"Okay," continued Gerry. "One study was done to compare neonatal neurobehavioral effects of Morphine or Meperidine administered to nursing mothers after they had undergone delivery by caesarean section. All this study showed, was that maternal administration of Meperidine caused breastfeeding infants to be somewhat less alert and responsive to speech than the infants of mothers administered Morphine (3). That's all. As regards other drugs such as Paracetamol and NSAID's—as I already told Mrs. Suk Ling, all these drugs can be administered in their normal dosages to breastfeeding women. No effects of these drugs on breastfeeding infants have ever been demonstrated. But chronic maternal ingestion of drugs such as benzodiazepines does sometimes cause some degree of sedation of their breastfeeding infants (1). One thing I didn't mention yet is the simple equation with which you can calculate the total amount of drug ingested by a baby in mothers' milk."

$$D_{(total\ dose)} = C_{(milk)} \text{ x } V_{(milk)}$$

- $D_{(total\ dose)}$ = total dose of drug ingested by the baby.
- $C_{(milk)}$ = concentration of drug in mothers' milk.
- $V_{(milk)}$ = volume of milk per feed (usually about 40-200 ml for a human baby).

Gerry continued, "This equation is so simple, that I find it impossible to resist doing a small calculation. Let's see what would happen if we gave Mrs. Suk Ling 10 mg Morphine intravenously, and then let her start breastfeeding her baby 20 minutes afterwards. How much Morphine would her baby ingest, and would this have a pharmacologically significant effect on her baby?"

- Weight of Mrs. Suk Ling's baby = 3.5 kg, and this hungry little baby drinks about 200 ml milk per feed.
- Weight of Mrs. Suk Ling = 54 kg.

**Morphine parameters (see Appendix)**
- $t_{1/2\alpha}$ = 4.4 min.
- $t_{1/2\beta}$ = 111 min.
- $V_d$ = 5.4 l/kg.
- $EC_{50}$ for postoperative analgesia = 0.015 mg/1.
- Dose of intravenous morphine = D = 10 mg = 10/54 = 0.185 mg/kg.
- Time between intravenous administration and beginning of breastfeeding = 20 min. This is a time period longer than $3 \times t_{1/2\alpha}$ = 3 x 4.4 = 13.2 min. Therefore distribution of Morphine is complete at this time.
- 20 minutes is a time much shorter than the plasma elimination half-life, so the maternal plasma Morphine concen-

Feeding time

tration at this time = $D/V_d$ = 0.185 / 5.4 = 0.034 mg/1. This is the plasma Morphine concentration resulting from a normal parenteral dose of Morphine in an adult that provides effective postoperative analgesia without causing significant respiratory depression.

- Assume Morphine concentrations in mother's milk and plasma are approximately equal.
- Mrs. Suk Ling's baby drinks 200 ml = 0.2 liter per feed. Accordingly, the total dose of Morphine ingested by her baby 20 minutes after she received a 10 mg intravenous dose of Morphine = 0.2 x 0.034 = 0.0068 mg.
- The baby of Mrs. Suk Ling weighs 3.5 kg, which means that the total oral dose of 0.0068 mg Morphine ingested by this baby = 0.0068/3.5 = 0.0019 mg/kg.
- The normal parenteral dose of Morphine for treating pain in infants up to six months of age is 0.05 to 0.1 mg/kg, and double this dosage is required for orally administered Morphine to provide effective analgesia. Accordingly, the baby of Mrs. Suk Ling will ingest an oral dose of Morphine in mother's milk that is 52 to 104 times lower than that required for a clinically significant analgesic effect without any respiratory depression.
- So even if morphine is present in mother's milk at a concentration somewhat higher than in plasma (actually the concentration of Morphine in mother's milk is 2.46 times greater than in plasma), there is only one conclusion possible. Letting Mrs. Suk Ling give breastfeeding 20 minutes after intravenous administration of 10 mg Morphine will cause no significant effect on her baby.

Bob was visibly impressed by this chain of reasoning, a fact expressed by his single guttural monosyllabic reaction, "Wow!" He and Gerry were so absorbed with their calculation, that they paid little attention to the operation, which lasted much shorter than expected. So just as Gerry finished his last sentence, Sluder called out, "Finished!" A typical ENT trick—maximum pain requiring maximum anesthesia, and then suddenly—finished!

Bob and Gerry knew what this meant. They knew full well it would take a while before this patient awoke. Bob administered Neostigmine and Atropine to antagonize the Rocuronium, Mrs. Suk Ling was ventilated for a short while with 100% oxygen to remove most of the Sevoflurane, and then switched over to manual ventilation. But she did not resume spontaneous respiration. She remained apneic. Sister Hörni (the anesthetic nurse), Bob, and Gerry stood in silence next to the patient. Every now and then Bob would squeeze the bag of the circle system in an almost desultory fashion, and during the subsequent expiration they observed the end tidal $CO_2$ ($ETCO_2$) concentration gradually increasing with each successive breath. Sluder and the scrub nurses departed for lunch, and an almost palpable hush descended upon and enveloped the room.

Finally, Gerry made a sound, "Humph. Tell me Bob, how fast do you think the $ETCO_2$ rises per minute during apnea? After all, you're ventilating this woman so minimally that you could say she's effectively apneic."

"Even so, her $SpO_2$ is above 96%,'replied Bob. "Strange... I see this happening every day, but I still don't quite understand how it's possible. I just accept it as a fact, because no-one ever talks about it."

"You lucky man, today is the day you will learn a pulmonary ventilation secret known only to a select few initiates. I will now induct you into the secrets of an old and almost forgotten pulmonary oxygenation technique called apneic oxygenation (4,5,6). I'll begin by asking my last question again—how fast does the $ETCO_2$ rise during apnea in an average adult? It's not a difficult question, because you can see it happening right in front of your eyes."

"The $ETCO_2$ of this woman is rising at a rate of about 0.3% per minute. But I really don't know the rate at which the $ETCO_2$ increases during apnea in other people," replied Bob.

"Your observation is correct for most adults. The $ETCO_2$ in most children and adults rises during apnea at a rate of 0.2% to 0.5% per minute (5), but rises more slowly during apnea in the aged than in the young, and rises more rapidly during hyper metabolic states such as cancer, inflammations, elevated temperature, or pregnancy. So tell me, what do you think the rate of rise of $ETCO_2$ has to do with oxygenation of the body?" asked Gerry with an unbearably smug look on his face. He was warming up to his subject, because during a long teaching career no-one had ever managed to answer this question."

Sister Hörni sighed. She knew this lesson had the potential to last a long time. So she went and got a magazine with the fascinating title, "Dressing Your Maltese Dog", out of her bag in the adjacent unused anesthetic induction room and sat down on a stool to read. She had heard these lessons before, and was in no mood to say, "Ooh, ah, fantastic." "Leave that to residents—that's what they're there for," she thought.

Bob was no exception to the rule. He was also unable to answer this question. So Gerry continued. "Listen well. This will really knock your socks off. It will change the way you look at some things. You ventilated this woman for several minutes with 100% oxygen before switching her to manual ventilation. This means her lungs were filled with 100% oxygen when you switched to manual ventilation. This woman is unconscious, comatose even, and accordingly her muscles are relaxed. This fact means her lung volume collapses down to her functional residual capacity (FRC) at the end of expiration. She weighs 54 kg, has a body length of about 165 cm, and is 25 years of age, which means her

FRC is about 2500 ml in a supine position. Now her $ETCO_2$ is increasing at a rate of 0.3% per minute, which means the fraction of $CO_2$ in her alveolar and pulmonary air increases by 0.3% per minute. This represents $CO_2$ streaming into her lungs from blood flowing through her alveolar capillaries. Now 0.3% of 2500 ml = 0.3 x 2500/100 = 7.5 ml, so every minute 7.5 ml of $CO_2$ enters this woman's lungs to elevate her $ETCO_2$ by 0.3% per minute."

Gerry paused to ask, "Are you still following me Bob?" Bob indicated he was all ears, so Gerry continued. "An average adult consumes oxygen at a rate of about 4 ml/kg/minute, which means this 54 kg woman will consume about 216 ml oxygen per minute. Blood continually flows through her oxygen filled lungs, and this blood absorbs the oxygen in her lungs at a rate of 216 ml/minute. But only 7.5 ml $CO_2$ is returned into her lungs per minute at the same time as this 216 ml oxygen is absorbed from her lungs each minute. The result is a negative pressure—more gas is removed from her lungs than is replaced. She is intubated, which means she has a good airway. Furthermore, a continuous source of oxygen is attached to her endotracheal tube, replenishing the oxygen absorbed by blood, and acting as a continuous supply of oxygen for her body. So her apneic body actually sucks oxygen into her lungs through the anesthetic system and endotracheal tube. This is how this effectively apneic woman is oxygenated. This is apneic oxygenation."

"So that explains this, and other similar situations," was Bob's reply. "In other words—first fill the lungs with oxygen, ensure a patent airway and a supply of oxygen, and you've got apneic oxygenation. Wow! I like it!"

"Yair," drawled Gerry, "and now you can tell me how long you can permit apneic oxygenation before people lose consciousness due to hypercarbia."

Bob's feeling of elation evaporated abruptly. "You mean you can calculate that too?"

"Yep! Look at this table of the effects of different levels of acute changes of arterial $CO_2$ ($P_aCO_2$) (Table 7.1)."

**Table 7.1**

Arterial carbon dioxide pressure and levels of consciousness (7-13)

| $P_aCO_2$ (mmHg) | $P_aCO_2$ (kPa) | Mental effects |
|---|---|---|
| 15< | 2< | All people unconscious |
| 20 | 2.7 | EEG slowing in 50% of people |
| 30 | 4 | Abnormal mental function in 50% of people & tetany |
| **35-45** | **4.5-6** | **NORMAL $P_aCO_2$** |
| >55 | >7 | Increasingly abnormal mental function |
| >75 | >10 | Increasing chance of loss of consciousness |
| >150 | >20 | All people unconscious & surgical anesthesia |
| >300 | >40 | Increasing chance of death |

Bob looked in wonder at the table. He had never seen this table anywhere before. Gerry was proud of this table—it was a product of much literature study. "Now Bob, the ETCO2 in percent is practically equal to the ETCO2 in kPa, because one standard atmosphere = 760 mmHg = 101.3 kPa, which is why gas partial pressures expressed as kPa can also be expressed as percentages of one atmosphere. Furthermore, arterial PCO2 ($P_aCO_2$) is always higher than the ETCO2, otherwise $CO_2$ simply would not diffuse out of blood into the lungs. This difference is about 0.2 to 0.5 kPa in young and healthy people, while in people with lung diseases this difference can be as much as 1.5 kPa. Do you follow me up till now Bob?"

"All clear," replied Bob.

Gerry continued. "Using all these data, we can now calculate the time it will take Mrs. Suk Ling to lose consciousness due to $CO_2$ accumulation during the apnea you induced with the anesthetic drugs you administered. Let's assume for the sake of simplicity that the $ETCO_2$ of this healthy young woman is about equal to her $P_aCO_2$. Her $ETCO_2$ at the start of apnea was 4.5%, and the $ETCO_2$ at which she has a chance of losing consciousness is about 10% because she isn't used to hypercapnia. We know the rate of rise of her $ETCO_2$ is 0.3% per minute, which means that the time she can remain apneic before she has a chance of losing consciousness due to hypercapnia = (10-4.5)/0.3 = 5.5/0.3 = 18.3 minutes! Pretty good hey?"

Bob looked amazed. "Is this really true? I've never heard of this type of thing before."

"Yes it certainly is true. In fact apneic oxygenation used to be a standard technique of oxygenation during laryngeal surgery in the past. There is one report of a man who underwent a 53 minute period of apneic oxygenation for laryngeal surgery, at the end of which he had a $P_aCO_2$ of about 33 kPa (250 mmHg) (14). True, at this $P_aCO_2$ the hypercapnic, and undoubtedly very red and sweaty body of this man probably shook and shuddered with each hyperdynamic heartbeat, but he was alive although unconscious—you could even say he had developed into a new form of humankind—homo pulsans!"

Bob grinned at the term homo pulsans. He was impressed. He liked these terms. This was one of those obscure physiological facts he enjoyed learning. He looked at his watch—it was time for lunch. He suddenly remembered that the topically applied cocaine was certainly still active, which meant that even if the Alfentanil in her body were antagonized, Mrs. Suk Ling would feel no pain. So it was time for Naloxone, otherwise the hungry hoards frequenting the hospital restaurant would gobble the best food, leaving him with the left-overs. A small dose of Naloxone was just what Mrs. Suk Ling needed—she awoke and was brought to the recovery room. Sister Hörni, Gerry, and Bob departed for lunch in the restaurant. It was a good morning's work. They had earned their lunch and a rest.

# 8

# Short and long

"Why are we still here Bob? Why isn't this patient already in the recovery room?" asked Gerry in a querulous tone as Bob squeezed the bag yet again.

The young woman being manually ventilated by Bob was a Ms. Ondine, a fanatical hockey player who had torn a meniscus during an unfortunate sudden turn. She had demanded to undergo her arthroscopy under general anesthesia, a demand Doctor Abe Colles (the orthopedic surgeon), and Doctor Bob were only too happy to fulfill. Both had dry throats after the previous three patients who had undergone their arthroscopies under spinal anesthesia. These patients had required much reassurance from Bob, and had continually asked Colles all manner of questions about what they saw on the arthroscope monitor. A silent patient, and the possibility of normal conversation during an operation under general anesthesia seemed an attractive prospect at the time.

Anesthesia was induced with 20 mcg Sufentanil followed by 200 mg Propofol. A laryngeal mask was inserted and anesthesia maintained with controlled ventilation with a gas mixture of oxygen, air, and Sevoflurane. Abe Colles was an efficient and rapid orthopedic surgeon, and finished the necessary medial meniscectomy within 12 minutes. But Ms. Ondine gave no sign of starting to breathe spontaneously upon completion of the meniscectomy. Shortly afterwards, an increasingly impatient Colles went off to drink coffee, chatter, and complain about slow anesthesiologists with other colleagues in the coffee room. So it was that Bob and Sister Beatrix (the anesthetic nurse), were left alone in the operating theater with an unconscious and apneic patient. (Sister Beatrix was a normally cheerful, although restrained, older woman with curiously thick ankles, and a very upper class accent.) Bob and Beatrix remained alone in the operating theater, unspeaking, engulfed by a listless ennui. Every now and then Bob would squeeze the balloon just to see what the capnograph revealed, as well as to see if there was any hint of returning respiration. But all in vain—Ms. Ondine refused to breathe.

After about fifteen minutes, Doctor Gerry walked in the room and heard from Bob what was going on. He looked at the anesthetic chart. He remained silent as he leaned against the anesthetic machine, toying idly with a spinal needle while observing Bob, looking at the concentrations of Sevoflurane remaining in end-expired air, and the absence of respiration. He temporarily disconnected the expiratory limb of the anesthetic system so as to sniff the exhaled gases in a loud and demonstrative manner. Finally he spoke. "Why are we still here Bob? Why isn't this patient already in the recovery room?" asked Gerry in a querulous tone as Bob squeezed the bag yet again. "I look at this patient, I smell the Sevoflurane in the expired gas, and I'm inspired to paraphrase a passage in a Hindu holy book called the "Bhadaranyaka Upanisad":

*After the apex of the heart becomes luminous, the*
*life-breath pulls itself out of the body; sometimes though*
*the eye, the skull, or the laryngeal mask. When it pulls*
*out, the life-breath pulls out along with it all Sevoflu-*

*rane; and when the Sevoflurane-breath departs, all organs return to normal function. (1)*

"But aside from this pleasant little interlude for semi-theological paraphrasology—tell me why are we still here?"

"The reason is simple," replied Bob. "She just won't breathe."

"Ohhhhh... And why not?"

"I used a 20 mcg dose of Sufentanil which should have finished working by now. Last night I simulated the pharmacokinetics of several doses of Sufentanil at home, calculating the effect durations for different bolus doses. According to those simulations, the 20 mcg dose of Sufentanil I administered shouldn't cause any significant respiratory depression, or even provide any postoperative analgesia after about 10 minutes." Bob paused, looked at Gerry, saw a familiar expression, and groaned, "Don't tell me, I see it in your eyes, you're going to tell me it's all nonsense."

Gerry grinned mischievously, "Yes and no. Your simulations are quite correct for plasma concentrations of drugs. But people don't experience analgesia due to Sufentanil because their blood cells are pain free—they experience analgesia because extravascular nerve cells mediating analgesia are affected by Sufentanil. The same is also true for respiratory depression. So you should actually calculate the brain concentrations of Sufentanil."

The face of Beatrix suddenly became animated. Her expression of listless ennui disappeared as rapidly as a tourist's wallet on the Ramblas in Barcelona. She interrupted, "I believe you'll both be staying here a while. My relief hasn't come yet, and I'm dying for a cup of coffee. So if you don't mind I'll take my break now." With these words she walked out of the operating theater leaving Bob at the mercy of Gerry and the now inevitable lesson.

Bob also lusted after a cup of coffee. Even so, he knew now that natural forces such as a Gerry learning moment were unstoppable. He knew how to play this game, so he began, "How can I calculate the brain concentrations of Sufentanil, or those of any other anesthetic drugs? Are there any measurements of brain anesthetic drug concentrations?"

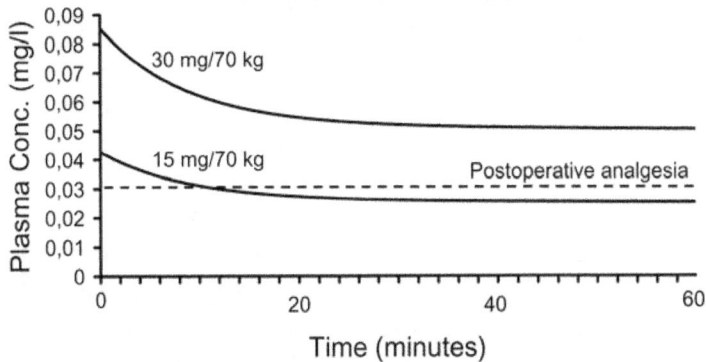

Figure 8.1: Plasma concentration-time curves resulting from two intravenous bolus doses of Methadone administered to average adults in relation to the plasma concentration at which most adults experience postoperative analgesia.

"No, there are no measurements of human brain drug concentrations that I know of for any drug. As I once said, there are very few people who would voluntarily want to undergo serial biopsies of their brains to determine brain drug diffusion constants—a sort of death by serial brain biopsy. Brrrr, doesn't bear thinking about! But back to business. Let's look at the example of Methadone. Methadone is an opiate with a distribution half-life of about 6 minutes, but an elimination half-life of about 35 hours. If you give a dose of about 15 mg Methadone, you see that distribution will cause the plasma Methadone concentration to drop below the analgesic plasma concentration after about 10 minutes. However, after administration of a higher 30 mg dose of Methadone, elimination causes the plasma Methadone concentration to fall below the analgesic level only after many hours. So the action of the lower dose is terminated by distribution, while the action of the higher dose is terminated by elimination (Figure 8.1)."

"You have the same with higher and lower doses of Sufentanil too," added Bob, "and that's why I used a low dose of Sufentanil."

"Hmmm," was Gerry's reaction to this fascinating snippet. He frowned, causing deep furrows to appear between his eyebrows, and continued. "Just a moment ago we were talking about the fact that opiates actually have to enter the brain to exert their action. So even though these calculations and simulations do seem to show that low dosages of these drugs may have a short duration of action when you only look at plasma concentrations, plasma and brain concentrations may actually be quite different. Immediately, and shortly after administration, the plasma concentrations of a drug are higher than the target organ tissue concentrations, and so drug diffuses out of the plasma into the target organ tissues. But as drug is distributed throughout the body, and eliminated from the plasma, plasma drug concentrations eventually decrease below target tissue drug concentrations, and so drug diffuses out of the tissues of the target organs back into the plasma. The volume of target tissue into which a drug must diffuse in order to exert an action can be described in single-, or multi-compartment pharmacokinetic models with an extra compartment called the effect compartment (see Figure 8.2). Furthermore, the speed of diffusion of drug into, or out of this effect compartment can be described with a mathematical exchange constant called the $k_{e0}$, and this constant has a half-life called the $t_{1/2}k_{e0}$ which is the half-life of the speed of equilibration of drug concentration between the plasma and the effect compartments. The shorter the $t_{1/2}k_{e0}$, the more rapidly a drug diffuses into, or out of the effect compartment, and vice versa. This half-life is calculated from the $k_{e0}$ with the formula below."

# Effect Compartment

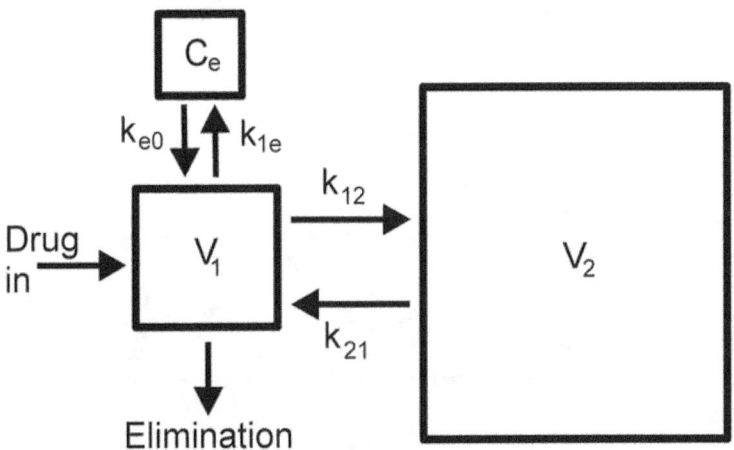

Figure 8.2: The relationship of the effect compartment ($C_e$) to the other compartments of a 2-compartment pharmacokinetic model.

$$t_{1/2}k_{e0} = 0.693 \,/\, k_{e0}$$

All this began to be a bit too much for Bob. His effect compartment caffeine concentration was well below the lower limit of the range considered compatible with normal function for anesthetic residents, and he was hungry. He desperately wanted caffeine and sweet carbohydrates in whatever form he could get them.

His eyes glazed, and he began to stare vacantly at nothing. Gerry recognized these signs and added, "Now we've finally come to the part where I can explain why knowledge of the existence, and implications of the $t_{1/2}k_{e0}$ will enrich your understanding of pharmacokinetics and pharmacodynamics. Such knowledge will improve your understanding about why some drugs act fast, while other drugs act slowly, why some drugs cease working rapidly, and others cease working slowly. And who knows, you may even become a better person for knowing these things."

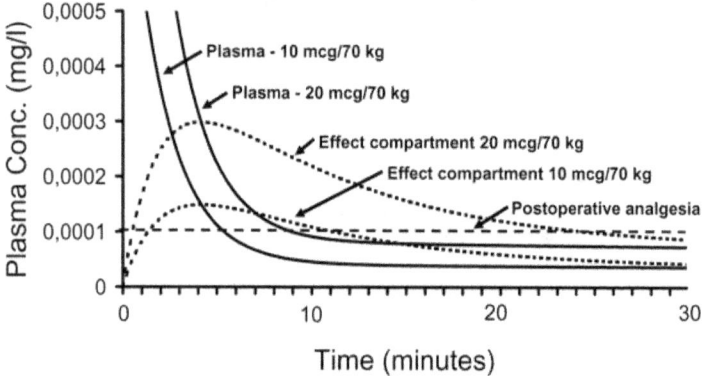

Figure 8.3: Plasma, and effect compartment concentrations of Sufentanil resulting from two different intravenous bolus doses administered to average adults. These are shown in relation to the plasma concentration of Sufentanil at which most adults experience postoperative analgesia.

This was something of mild interest to Bob. He aroused himself sufficiently to say in a voice that almost sounded convincingly enthusiastic. "I'm all ears."

Gerry continued, "Effect compartment concentrations can really only be calculated, not measured. So I've got some printouts of computer simulations illustrating the implications of the $t_{1/2}k_{e0}$.

I'll begin with a simulation of the effect compartment concentrations resulting from two doses of Sufentanil—a dose of 10 mcg and one of 20 mcg (see Figure 8.3). When you look at the graphs you see two things. Changes in Sufentanil effect compartment concentrations always lag several minutes behind the changes in plasma Sufentanil concentrations. This is not at all surprising when you consider that Sufentanil has a long $t_{1/2}k_{e0}$ of about 6 minutes, and like every other drug, must first diffuse into the effect compartment from plasma, and later diffuse out of the effect compartment back into the plasma. So when you look at the effect compartment concentrations of the 20 mcg Sufentanil dose you administered, you see that after achieving a peak concentration, Sufentanil effect compartment concentrations remain higher than the plasma concentrations for several minutes. This explains why your simulation of the plasma Sufentanil concentrations gave you illusory information about the duration of action of the 20 mcg dose of Sufentanil you administered to Ms. Ondine. Your simulation only showed that the plasma concentrations would only remain above postoperative the analgesic concentration for less than 10 minutes. But when you look at the effect compartment concentrations in this simulation, you see that the effect compartment concentrations of such a dose of Sufentanil will remain above the analgesic concentration somewhere up to 13 to 14 minutes after the plasma Sufentanil concentration has decreased below the analgesic concentration. Effect site concentrations of Sufentanil causing apnea are unknown. All that is known is that Sufentanil causes a dose-related respiratory depression at effect site concentrations above those needed for analgesia, and that this respiratory depression is enhanced by volatile anesthetic agents such as Sevoflurane. This is undoubtedly why Ms. Ondine is still apneic."

Bob looked at the simulation Gerry showed him, and understood what he had done. He nodded, and began. "Now I realize what is happening here. I also see on this simulation that if I want a drug to start working quickly, then I have to administer a larger bolus dose so that the concentration difference between the plasma and effect compartment is high enough to cause rapid diffusion of drug into the tissues of the effect compartment."

"Very good Bob. But that's not the only way to rapidly achieve therapeutic effect compartment concentrations. You can also administer drugs with a short $t_{1/2}k_{e0}$. Let's look at the example of opiates. I've made a simulation of the effects of 1 mg of a theoretical opiate (see Figure 8.4). In this simulation, I also simulated the changes in effect compartment concentrations resulting from the situation where this opiate has a $t_{1/2}k_{e0}$ of 1.1 minute, and for the situation where the $t_{1/2}k_{e0}$ is equal to 6 minutes. This simulation clearly shows that for the same dosage and plasma concentration changes, that the effect compartment concentrations and the resulting clinical effects differ according to the $t_{1/2}k_{e0}$. In the situation with a short $t_{1/2}k_{e0}$, the effect compartment concentrations are higher, change synchronously with, and are nearly equal to the plasma concentrations. This is not the situation when the $t_{1/2}k_{e0}$ is 6 minutes. Here the effect compartment concentrations rise slowly, the peak effect compartment concentrations are lower, and lag minutes behind those in the plasma. The conclusions are evident. So tell me Bob, what have you learned from these simulations?"

Bob fished his notebook out of a pocket and looked up the tables of pharmacokinetic and pharmacodynamic parameters. He was beginning to get enthusiastic about the implications of the $t_{1/2}k_{e0}$ in relation to drug usage. "Now I understand. You always have to consider the $t_{1/2}k_{e0}$ in relation to the pharmacokinetic parameters, because clinical utility is determined by the relationship between pharmacodynamic and pharmacokinetic profiles. So in the situation of opiates, I could make the following list."

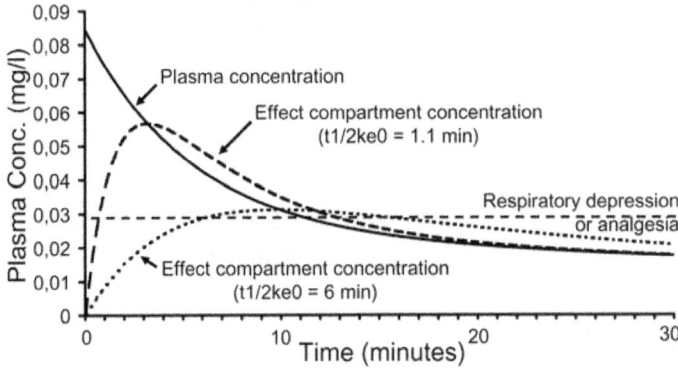

Figure 8.4: Plasma concentration-time curve of a single intra-venous bolus dose of an imaginary opiate in relation to the effect compartment concentration associated with respiratory depression or analgesia for that opiate. Note the differences in effect compartment concentration curves, and hence differences in clinical effect resulting from a short versus a long $t_{1/2}k_{e0}$. Such differences in $t_{1/2}k_{e0}$ determine the clinical usage of drugs administered as intravenous boluses during anesthesia.

- For very short operations, I would use an opiate such as Alfentanil or Remifentanil, because each has a short $t_{1/2}k_{e0}$ as well as a short elimination half-life.
- For long operations, use either an infusion of a short acting opiate such as Remifentanil, or use an opiate with a longer elimination half-life where the length of the $t_{1/2}k_{e0}$ is relatively unimportant.
- If a patient under general anesthesia has a sudden extreme reaction to the pain of an operation, administration of an opiate with a short $t_{1/2}k_{e0}$ is more appropriate because it will act faster than an opiate with a long $t_{1/2}k_{e0}$. So you could say that Fentanyl and Sufentanil are drugs you give

in anticipation of expected responses to painful stimuli because of their relatively long $t_{1/2}k_{e0}$'s, while Alfentanil or Remifentanil are drugs you can give in reaction to responses to painful stimuli because of their short $t_{1/2}k_{e0}$'s.

"And...," continued Bob, "the concept of the $t_{1/2}k_{e0}$ means in the case of intravenously administered hypnotic and induction agents, that the following considerations apply."

- Clinical doses of induction agents with a short $t_{1/2}k_{e0}$ will usually exert a hypnotic effect within one circulation time, because such drugs diffuse rapidly into their effect compartments.
- It takes longer for drugs with a long $t_{1/2}k_{e0}$, such as Midazolam, to exert a hypnotic effect, because it takes time for such drugs to diffuse into their effect compartments.
- The same considerations also apply to hypnotic agents administered by intravenous infusions.

Gerry nodded, "So Bob, you're beginning to understand what it's all about. One day soon you'll be able to call yourself a real specialist in pharmacokinetics and pharmacodynamics. Now for a little extra supplement to the kinetic and dynamic concepts we've been discussing. The pharmacokinetic simulations I've shown you here are wonderful products of complex calculations, but they always show a peak plasma drug concentration at zero seconds after injection." Gerry's back straightened, his index finger pointed upwards, and small foam flecks appeared at the corners of his mouth as he stated in a stern voice, "But this is a lie! A peak plasma drug concentration at zero seconds after intravenous injection is an anatomical and physiological impossibility! I will recite a small list to tell you why."

- After injecting a drug into a vein, the drug is initially present only in the vein.
- The flow of blood in the vein transports the drug-laden blood to the right heart.
- The heart pumps this drug-laden blood through the lungs into the left heart.
- The left heart pumps drug-laden blood into the arterial system in which it is transported to all parts of the body.
- This means that the time to peak drug plasma concentration in arterial or venous blood in any part of the body is dependent upon circulation times to those parts of the body.

"All this means no drug can ever achieve peak arterial or venous drug concentrations at zero time. It always takes time for a peak plasma concentration to be achieved, which means it always takes time for an intravenously administered drug to act." Gerry added in conclusion of his sermon. "These are physiological facts that must always be taken into account during the first few minutes of the administration of any drug. Now that's enough learning for one day. Hey, look at this! Ms. Ondine has finally started breathing, although she's still not awake. Okay, one out of two is not so bad. Even so, why isn't she awake yet Bob?"

"Well Gerry, I think she's basically catatonic with boredom. She doesn't really want to learn anything about pharmacokinetics and pharmacodynamics. A real shame. I'm sure millions of people would love to broaden their intellectual horizons, and enrich their lives with such valuable knowledge." Bob muttered a "Tsk, tsk," shook his head and proceeded to remove the tape holding the laryngeal mask in place. He did this with verve and vigor, as well as to the accompaniment the sound of tape tearing painfully loose from delicate facial skin. The hands of Ms. Ondine rose by reflex to her mouth, her eyes opened, she drew a deep breath, and she opened her mouth—she was awake. Bob reacted predictably and pragmatically—he quickly removed the laryngeal mask. "Ah, Ms. Ondine, you're awake! The operation is finished. We'll bring you to the recovery room." "And," thought Bob, "afterwards I can sit down and drink a cup of strong coffee as well as eat one of those delicious sausage rolls one of the nurses was talking about." Gerry looked approvingly upon all these things. He saw that Bob was a pragmatist, a fast learner with a sense of proportion and humor, growing in professional stature and ability. This was going well. But now it was time for important matters—coffee.

# 9

# The arterial reality of infusions

Mr. Dingleberry was a wiry, unintelligent, little man whose sallow skin was decorated with multiple tattoos of snakes, dragons, Celtic symbols, and naked women in fascinating poses. He had been arrested the night before after the police gave chase to an evidently drunken man riding a motor scooter, only catching him after a wild chase through small streets and alleys, in one of which he finally scraped a lamppost, fell, and broke his leg. Mr. Dingleberry was destined for a police cell, but with a very evidently broken leg, he first needed repairing. Accordingly, the police had called an ambulance to bring him to Saint Elders Hospital, where he was admitted.

The following afternoon, a somewhat recalcitrant, sober, but very hung-over Mr. Dingleberry was brought to the operating theater for an operation on his nasty tibia-plateau fracture. Doctor Bob read the clinical notes and spoke with him. Mr. Dingleberry was a chain-smoker, a heavy drinker, and had chronic bronchitis that he treated with a most interesting remedy—smoking even more cigarettes. "I always breathe much easier after I smoke heavy cigarettes without filters," he said. "I wasn't feeling too well this morning, so I smoked a few in my bed before the nurses made their first rounds." Bob was always "delighted" with this type of patient, and after hearing Dingleberry's juicily fruity cough, decided spinal anesthesia was the most appropriate anesthetic technique. His choice of anesthesia was greeted with wholehearted disapproval from Mr. Dingleberry. Even so, Bob insisted this was the best form of anesthesia for this operation in this clinical situation.

Cries of "Ow, ow, owwww....," together with hyperextension of Dingleberry's back, followed by a short vasovagal cardiac arrest during administration of the spinal anesthetic, rapidly convinced Bob that Dingleberry was not only violently allergic to good sense and policemen, but also allergic to needles, and possibly even to anesthesiologists (this latter is a rare and almost unheard of phenomenon). He and Sister Cybele the anesthetic nurse quickly laid Dingleberry flat on the table, upon which Cybele administered a rapid and firm precordial thump, so restoring normal sinus rhythm.

Cybele remarked, "Why is it that it's always men with tattoos that go all vasovagal with drips and spinal needles. It seems like the more tattoos, the greater the chance of a vasovagal attack. Weaklings!" Cybele was a notorious man-hater, a stern and terrifyingly capable anesthetic nurse—especially harsh with residents—giving as a reason, "They're here to learn, they're here to work, and they have to be disciplined for their own good." She was in a bad mood because she was working with Doctor Bob, a male resident, and had not yet seen Doctor Gerry, her favorite anesthesiologist, that morning.

"I haven't a clue why tattooed men do that either, but it's something you see a lot," responded Bob as he thought. "Must be spinal reflexes. After all, this man has the intelligence of a demented rabbit."

Dr. Percy Pott interrupted what otherwise might have developed into an interesting and profound discussion about the physiological differences between men and women, as well as factors that might drive men to alcoholism and into tattoo parlors. "Can I start now?" Pott was a pleasant man, an efficient orthopedic surgeon, quite good at traumatology, especially in ankle surgery.

"Please do," replied Bob.

The broken leg was quickly disinfected with iodine and draped. Soon afterwards, typical sounds of surgical contentment were heard across the sterile drape separating surgical and anesthetic worlds: instruments were requested and given, the surgeon monopolized the conversation with his weak jokes and boring stories, while every now and then the buzzing of diathermy was heard. All was well in surgeon territory, but this was not the case on the anesthetic side of the sterile drapes. After a total of 10 mg intravenous Midazolam, Dingleberry was a little calmer than before, no longer sweating, but still complaining and moaning about everything. Bob decided to sedate him with a Propofol infusion, so that everyone could have a bit of peace. An infusion pump was attached to his drip, and Propofol infused at a rate of 200 mg/hr. Dingleberry fell asleep about 10 to 15 minutes after starting the Propofol infusion, a state of consciousness heralded by hideous sounds comparable to a berserk chainsaw—the Propofol infusion had revealed another of Dingleberry's charming attributes—he snored horribly. Bob shook him by the shoulder every now and then to awaken him whenever the snoring was too loud or too awful to bear. Otherwise relative peace and contentment was present on both sides of the sterile drapes. The operation lasted two and a half hours, and Dingleberry was awake a few minutes afterwards. His first question was predictable, and received with the usual smiles, "When are you going to start the operation?"

Gerry walked into the operating theater just as Bob and Cybele started bringing Dingleberry to the recovery room. He nodded to Pott in a friendly manner; they had worked with each other for many years. Each respected the abilities of the other, and they even got along quite well. Gerry said, "Ah Bob, you're finished. Just a minute while I have a quick look at the anesthetic chart... Hmmmm... Okay, I'll stay here to discuss some things with Percy, while you go to the recovery room with Cybele. I'll also order the next patient."

"Okay', Bob answered, and they left. But when Bob and Cybele came back, the operating theater was empty of everyone but for Gerry and Pott. "Where's the next patient?" asked Bob.

"I've just heard that the lift is stuck, so the next patient will be delayed until it's fixed," was Gerry's response. "Percy why don't you go and have a cup of coffee, gossip with your colleagues, catch up with your administration—something I believe surgeons of all sorts love doing—or do whatever orthopedic surgeons do whenever they have a bit of unexpected spare time. Bob and I are going to talk about some of the fascinating aspects of pharmacokinetics and pharmacodynamics revealed by the anesthetic administered to Mr. Dingleberry while we're waiting for the lift to be fixed."

Bob also desperately wanted a cup of coffee. His effect compartment caffeine concentration was rapidly falling below that compatible with life and normal function in an anesthetic resident, but he knew an unstoppable learning moment was at hand. So he was pleasantly relieved to hear Gerry say, "Come on Bob, surgeons can go to the coffee room where they can drink coffee with their own sort. We'll go to my room where I've got some really good coffee, as well as some totally irresponsible biscuits. Cybele, could you call us when the next patient arrives?"

"Okay. Enjoy yourselves." and with this short response, Cybele also left for the coffee room in glad anticipation of coffee, a newspaper and a gossip, happy in the knowledge it would take some time to repair the aged lifts gracing Saint Elders Hospital.

Seated with mugs of steaming hot coffee and biscuits from Gerry's private stores before them, Gerry began, "How did it go with the Propofol infusion you administered to the unsavory Mr. Dingleberry?"

"Good," was the response, "was there anything particularly special about how it went?"

"As far as normal anesthetic practice went—nothing. But how did you calculate the intravenous infusion rate for this patient?"

"I didn't," replied Bob. "I just used an infusion rate that seems to work with most people."

"So how would you calculate the intravenous infusion rate otherwise?"

Bob had once prepared himself for this very question, so his answer was almost instantaneous. "The equation is as follows."

$$Q = C_{ss} \times Cl$$

- $Q$ = infusion rate expressed mg/kg/hr.
- $C_{ss}$ = steady state plasma concentration expressed as mg/1.
- $Cl$ = plasma clearance expressed as 1/kg/hr.

"Very good," was Gerry's response. "At least you know the formula. Now calculate the expected plasma Propofol concentration you would have achieved with your infusion of 200 mg per hour. Mr. Dingleberry is small and skinny, so let's say his weight is 60 kg."

"Okay. Let's see," said Bob. "This is easy. What a simple calculation!" He put his calculation in the form of a list (see the appendix for drug data).

- Body weight of Dingleberry = 60 kg.

- Infusion rate = 200 mg/hr = 200 / 60 = 3.33 mg/kg/hr.
- Propofol plasma clearance = 3.55 1/kg/hr.
- Plasma Propofol concentration due to this infusion = $C_{ss}$ = Q / Cl = 3.33 / 3.55 = 0.94 mg/1.
- Sleep concentration of Propofol = 2 mg/1.

"Er..." remarked Bob upon looking at these results. "If this calculation is correct, then Dingleberry shouldn't have been asleep at all. But he was asleep, although we were able to arouse him quite easily by shaking his shoulder and speaking loudly in his ear. Are you sure these pharmacokinetic and pharmacodynamic parameters are correct?"

"Oh they're correct, but your thinking isn't," was Gerry's blunt response. "What you told me about the reactions of Mr. Dingleberry clearly indicate his level of consciousness was at a level of sedation equivalent to a Ramsay score of 3. In other words he was asleep, but reacted to shaking his shoulder as well as to loud speech. Some research has been done into the relationship between Ramsay score and the effect compartment concentrations of Propofol (see Table 9.1)."

"What you didn't consider was the fact that the steady state plasma concentration for sleep that you cited was for unconsciousness together with minimal response to pain—something quite different to the level of sedation you described. Minimal pain reaction only occurs at a Ramsay score of 5 and above. Now if you look at this table you see that Mr. Dingleberry's effect compartment Propofol concentration must have been somewhere in the region of 0.6 mg/1, a concentration somewhat lower than that which you calculated."

"I understand," interrupted Bob enthusiastically, "but pharmacokinetic and pharmacodynamic parameters are only average values for sometimes quite different study populations, so the difference between the level I calculated and the reality is very likely within this variation. Furthermore, Mr. Dingleberry is a heavy drinker, which means he is used to general anesthetic drugs such as alcohol, so he probably needs a higher Propofol concentration than most people for an equivalent level of sedation. In other words, this calculation elegantly describes why the level of consciousness of Dingleberry was at the Ramsay score of 3 that I observed."

**Table 9.1**

Relation of Ramsay Score to Propofol Effect Compartment concentrations

| Ramsay Score | Definition | Propofol effect compartment concentration (mg/l) |
|---|---|---|
| 0 | Normal consciousness | 0 |
| 1 | Agitated, restless and anxious | |
| 2 | Awake, cooperative, tolerates ventilation | 0.25 (1) |
| 3 | Asleep, but cooperative – opens eyes in response to shaking, movement, or loud speech | 0.6 (1) |
| 4 | Deep sedation – does not open eyes in reponse to loud speech or movement, but does react promptly to pain | 1.0 (1) |
| 5 | Anesthesia – minimal reaction to pain only | 2.0 (1) |
| 6 | Coma – no reaction to pain at all | 2.28 (2,3) |

"I wouldn't get too excited if I was you," said Gerry. "A general rule for constant rate infusions is that it takes at least three to four elimination half-lives before the plasma concentration of an infused drug achieves a true steady state plasma concentration. In the case of Propofol, the elimination half-life is about 55 minutes for a two-compartment model, which means it would have taken about three to four hours before Dingleberry's plasma Propofol concentration achieved the level you calculated. Three to four hours is rather longer than the operation on Dingleberry lasted, and a lot longer than the 10 to 15 minutes you told me it took before he was sedated to a Ramsay score of 3. You can see this in the simulation I've made of the situation of a 200 mg/hr Propofol perfusion (figure 9.1). I should add here, that at these time-scales the $t_{1/2}k_{e0}$ of 2.9 minutes for Propofol is insignificant, and so the plasma and effect concentrations are just about equal. What do you make of all this Bob?"

"Then why did Dingleberry fall asleep so rapidly? Other people also observe that most patients fall asleep 10 to 15 minutes after starting a Propofol infusion at a rate of 200 mg/hr. What everyone else and I observe at this perfectly standard Propofol infusion rate is true. So this means either the pharmacokinetic parameters are incorrect, or you applied the equations incorrectly."

"The pharmacokinetic parameters are perfectly standard parameters for single bolus injections of Propofol. Nothing incorrect there. The mathematical two-compartment model equations for drug infusions are also perfectly correct and perfectly accurate. The use of these equations is also correct." Gerry then put his hand over his heart, looked theatrically towards the heavens with a loathsomely smug expression on his face, while declaiming loudly, "This is all true! Believe me, I'm a doctor."

Bob groaned inwardly at the sight of such appallingly awful theater. "So what's going on then? I have a sneaking suspicion there's another aspect to this problem you haven't told me."

"You're quite right. Here we have a situation where observation and theory do not seem to correspond. This means we have to either massage the facts to fit the theory—an act of loathsome depravity known as a Procrustean crime—or we construct a new theory. But this is not necessary, because theory and practice do correspond in this model, only we're applying the theory inappropriately."

Bob took another sip of the coffee Gerry had given him, noted from his tachycardia that it must contain almost toxic levels of caffeine, was gladdened by the thought his coronary arteries were evidently in good condition, leaned back, and looked expectantly at Gerry, who continued, "What you, and just about everyone does is to use venous plasma drug concentrations. Nearly all drug pharmacokinetic parameters, and all these equations, accurately describe drug pharmacokinetics based upon measurements of venous plasma drug concentrations. You may well ask why venous blood sampling is used to determine drug pharmacokinetic parameters? The answer is that venous blood sampling to derive pharmacokinetic parameters is an easy, safe, and simple way of repeatedly obtaining many blood samples. But venous blood is what comes out of the tissue capillary beds of the body. Venous blood drug concentrations do not tell you concentrations of drugs actually going into tissue capillary beds—that is determined by arterial blood drug concentrations. And venous plasma drug concentrations are quite different from arterial plasma drug concentrations in the first 5-8 minutes after bolus drug injections, as well as for some time after starting drug infusions (4,5,6,7). So let's make a calculation for the case of Mr. Dingleberry based on arterial Propofol plasma drug concentrations—an explanation based on physiology and pharmacodynamics."

"As if I couldn't guess you wouldn't have a physiological explanation," grumbled Bob.

"I know, I know, but I can't help myself. So here it is in the form of a list," replied Gerry.

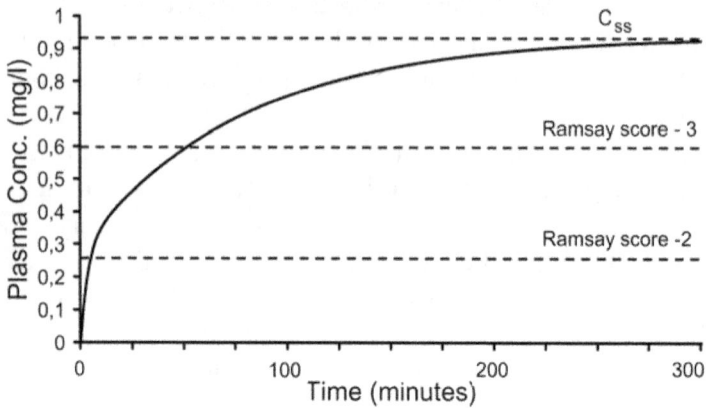

Figure 9.1: Change of plasma Propofol concentration with time as a result of a Propofol infusion administered at a constant rate of 200 mg/hr to an average adult. The plasma Propofol concentrations are shown in relation to the desired Css and the effect compartment concentrations associated with different Ramsay sedation scores.

- Rate of Propofol infusion administered to Mr. Dingleberry = 200 mg/hr = 200/60 = 3.33 mg/min.
- This constant drug infusion mixed with the venous blood returning to Mr. Dingleberry's heart at a flow equivalent to the cardiac output.
- Propofol is quite fat soluble, so blood and plasma concentrations are approximately equal.
- Approximate cardiac output of Mr. Dingleberry while more or less at rest after 10 g of i.v. Midazolam = 5 1/min.
- During the first 2 minutes of a Propofol infusion, Propofol is absorbed into lung tissue (8), and only after equili-

brium is achieved between lung and blood Propofol does the full 3.33 mg/min Propofol enter the left heart.

- This means that after about two minutes, the Propofol concentration in blood pumped into the arteries by the left heart = [Infusion Rate] / [Cardiac Output] = 3.33/5 = 0.666 mg/l.
- Arteries transport blood with this concentration of Propofol to the brain.
- Brain tissue, or effect compartment Propofol concentration is equal to the plasma concentration after 3 to 4 times the $t_{1/2}k_{e0}$ of Propofol (2.9 minutes). So the effect compartment Propofol concentration is about equal to the plasma Propofol concentration after 9 to 12 minutes.
- Add the time of equilibration of Propofol with lung tissue. So the total time needed to achieve a brain Propofol concentration capable of generating a Ramsay sedation score of 3 is = 2 plus 9 to 12 minutes = 11 to 14 minutes.

"In other words," continued Gerry, "this method of calculation yields an almost spookily correct arterial plasma Propofol concentration, as well as explaining why Mr. Dingleberry was sedated to a Ramsay score of 3 in such a short time."

Bob was impressed. This was the way to view pharmacokinetics and pharmacodynamics! His expression manifested a sincere look of approval, even as he laughed, "Gerry, why don't you change your name to Procrustes? Fudging the cardiac output as you just did to achieve a spookily correct result like this is an achievement worthy of Procrustes himself!" He continued, "However, I understand the principle, and can see that this principle is applicable to a lot of clinical situations. If a person is anxious and has a high cardiac output, then you will need a higher infusion rate for the same drug effect. And if a person has a low cardiac output, either due to age or disease, then you can use a lower infusion rate to achieve the same effect."

Bob began to warm to this chain of reasoning. "When you think about it, administration of anesthetic vapors can also be treated in exactly the same way as intravenous infusions, only the drugs enter the circulation through the lungs instead of being injected directly into a blood vessel. So people with a high cardiac output due to anxiety, fever, high output sepsis, youth, or whatever, need higher vapor concentrations. On the other hand, people with low cardiac outputs such as the elderly, or those with severe heart disease, hypovolemia, etc, need much lower vapor concentrations for the same effect. Wow, this is good." Bob looked really pleased. Theory and physiology were united into a usable clinical paradigm! Then he appeared to realize something, and asked, "But what about when you want the drug that you administer by infusion to act almost immediately, as in the situations of inotropics or total intravenous anesthesia?"

"Then you need a loading dose to rapidly elevate the plasma concentrations of the infused drug," replied Gerry. "A loading dose is simply an extra dose of the same drug administered at the beginning of an infusion to rapidly raise the plasma drug concentration to, or above the desired concentration, and to hopefully keep it at this concentration. There are all manner of systems of calculating such a dose. One method is the old Boyes method, where the loading dose is calculated with the formula below."

$$D_{(loading)} = C_{ss} \times V_c$$

"If we simulate such a loading dose together with the 200 mg/hr infusion we gave to Mr. Dingleberry, we get the curve in Figure 9.2. Let's calculate the Boyes loading dose for the situation of Mr. Dingleberry."

- Desired plasma Propofol concentration ($C_{ss}$) to achieve a Ramsay score of 3 = 0.6 mg/1 (Table 9.1).
- Propofol central compartment volume = $V_c$ = 0.63 l/kg (see Appendix).

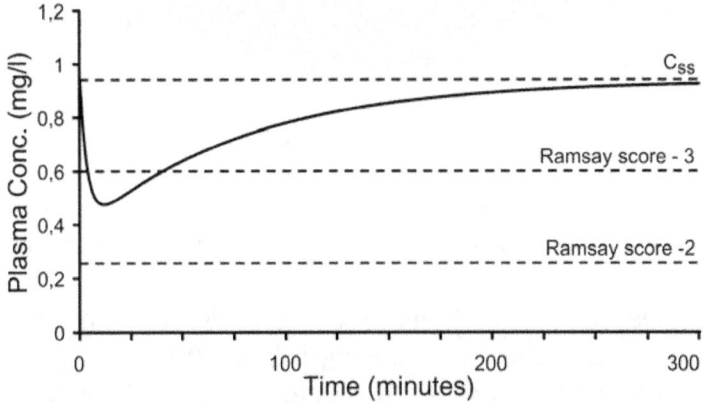

Figure 9.2: This is a plasma concentration-time curve for Propofol. It is exactly the same situation as in Figure 9.1 where the Propofol is administered at a constant rate of 200 mg/hr. The difference is that a Boyes loading dose has been administered at the beginning of the infusion. The effect of this loading dose is that the plasma Propofol concentration is initially at the desired $C_{ss}$, but rapidly drops below this level until steady state is achieved.

- Desired Boyes loading dose = $D_{(loading)}$ = $C_{ss}$ x $V_c$ = 0.6 x 0.63 = 0.378 mg/kg.
- Body weight of Mr. Dingleberry = 60 kg.
- Therefore the Boyes loading dose for Mr. Dingleberry = 60 x 0.378 = 22.68 mg.

"With this loading dose, the venous plasma Propofol concentrations will drop below the desired venous plasma concentration very rapidly. However, we wouldn't worry about that for most infusions, unless the arterial plasma Propofol concentration is lower than that desired. Those obsessed by a desire to maintain venous plasma drug concentrations at levels above, or equal to the desired levels, can use the Mitenko & Ogilvie method to calculate a loading dose with the formula below."

$$\mathbf{D_{(loading)} = C_{ss} \ x \ V_d}$$

"Let's amuse ourselves by calculating the desired Mitenko and Ogilvie loading dose for the insalubrious Mr. Dingleberry."

- Desired plasma Propofol concentration ($C_{ss}$) to achieve a Ramsay score of 3 = 0.6 mg/1 (Table 9.1).
- Propofol volume of distribution = $V_d$ = 4.7 l/kg (Appendix).
- Desired Mitenko and Ogilvie loading dose = $D_{(loading)}$ = $C_{ss}$ x $V_d$ = 0.6 x 4.7 = 2.82 mg/kg.
- Body weight of Mr. Dingleberry = 60 kg.
- Therefore the Mitenko and Ogilvie loading dose for Mr. Dingleberry = 60 x 2.82 = 169.2 mg.

This is a full anesthetic induction dose of Propofol, and as such is a bit extreme for a loading dose intended only to induce and maintain a Ramsay score of no more than 3.

If we simulate such a loading dose together with the 200 mg/hr infusion you administered to Mr. Dingleberry, we get the curve in Figure 9.3.

"Even so, you can see from Figure 9.3 that this is a very efficient method of administering a loading dose that will maintain venous drug concentrations at a desired level. One problem is that it is a relatively large loading dose, which means that sometimes you may cause toxic effects, or myocardial depression with some drugs. Are you still following me Bob?"

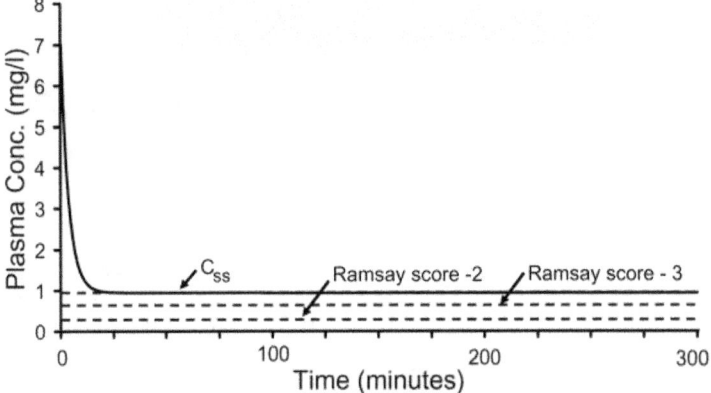

Figure 9.3: This is a plasma concentration-time curve for Propofol. It is exactly the same situation as in Figure 9.1 where the Propofol is administered at a constant rate of 200 mg/hr. The difference is that a Mitenko & Ogilvie loading dose has been administered at the beginning of the infusion. The effect of this loading dose is that the plasma Propofol concentration is much higher than the desired $C_{ss}$ and never drops below the desired $C_{ss}$.

"Yes, it's all fairly clear. But what about other techniques of administering loading doses? A lot of hospitals administer anesthesia with a total intravenous anesthesia (TIVA) technique, simultaneously administering opiates, hypnotics, and muscle relaxants with separate intravenous infusions to provide the three basic components of general anesthesia: unconsciousness, muscle relaxation, and analgesia. It's easy to calculate the steady state infusion rate, but, as you've just made abundantly clear, the main problem is calculating the loading dose. So are there other systems and methods?" asked Bob.

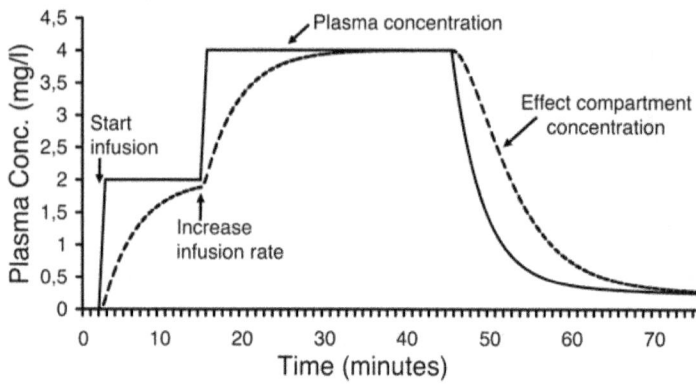

Figure 9.4: Theoretical possible plasma concentration-time curve for Propofol administered by a modern computer controlled TIVA pump with effect compartment steering. As can be seen, such modern TIVA pumps can administer step-wise increments in plasma drug concentrations, which are followed by changes in effect compartment concentrations. These are active processes controlled by the perfusor pump. However, reduction of plasma and effect compartment drug concentrations is a passive process set in action by reducing the infusion rate, or by stopping drug administration. Drug concentrations then decline due to plasma elimination, as well as exchange of drug between other compartments and the central compartment.

"There is actually a veritable plethora of loading dose systems: systems with multiple boluses, systems with stepped infusion rates, systems with effect compartment concentration targeting, computer controlled electronic infusion pumps, etc, etc. Many are even very good. For practical clinical work in modern hospitals, the best method of applying a total intravenous anesthetic technique, or intravenous infusions of most anesthetic drugs is to use modern computer controlled intravenous infusion pumps incorporating algorithms with pharmacokinetic-effect compartment modeling to control drug infusion rates. They are in general really very good. They save you a lot of thinking and a lot of work. Your brain won't be anywhere near as tired at the end of the day. However, if you don't have the luxury of possessing these computer controlled pumps, then you have to do it the old-fashioned way. Administer a Boyes loading dose followed by extra small doses as needed. Are you following me Bob? You look a bit bemused."

"Yes, it's all clear to me, but it's a lot to digest in one session. Okay, the considerations of starting and maintaining a drug infusion are obvious. Even your iconoclastic opinion about arterial versus venous drug concentrations is evident and proven by clinical practice. But how long after stopping an intravenous infusion does it take before the concentration of a drug administered by an infusion decreases to insignificance? Can I predict the rate of decline with the distribution and elimination half lives?"

"Good question Bob, but there is no really simple answer for practical clinicians. In general, for very short infusions, you can predict the rate of plasma drug concentration decline by considering the total administered dose as a single bolus dose—so the rate of decline can be predicted with bolus dose distribution and elimination pharmacokinetics. However, the longer a drug infusion is continued, the more the body is saturated with drug at that concentration. So when the drug infusion is stopped, the rate of decline of plasma drug concentration is not only determined by the rate of drug clearance from the plasma compartment, but is also determined to a large degree by the rate drug diffuses from the deep, or peripheral compartment into the plasma from which it is eliminated. In this situation the rate of decline is quite different from that given by the elimination half-life for bolus drug administration. This is actually the idea of the context sensitive half-time, which is defined as the time taken for the plasma concentration of a drug to decrease by 50% after stopping an intravenous infusion of that drug. In this case, the context is the duration of the drug infusion."

"An interesting idea," responded Bob. "But as a practical clinician, how do I use context sensitive half-times in my daily anesthetic practice?"

"I was afraid you might ask that Bob. The concept of the context sensitive half time is very powerful when simulating intravenous drug infusions with computers, or when programmed into computer controlled intravenous drug infusion pumps, but useless for people without these things. There is only a general rule to guide you as a practical clinician—the context sensitive half-time of a drug is always shorter than the intravenous bolus plasma elimination half-life of that drug, regardless of the infusion duration. In practice, this means that anesthesiologists in well-financed modern hospitals use computer controlled intravenous infusion pumps to administer total intravenous anesthesia, or other drug infusions, as well as to determine how and when to stop an intravenous infusion. As I said earlier, modern intravenous perfusor pumps designed for anesthetic purposes using pharmacokinetic-pharmacodynamic modeling do this extremely well. Figure 9.4 gives an illustration of how such a modern perfusor pump can automatically adjust the infusion speed to achieve stepped infusions at multiple desired plasma, or effect compartment drug concentrations within a given time. Furthermore such perfusor pumps are also programmed to use pharmacokinetic-pharmacodynamic modeling to stop intravenous drug infusions at the appropriate times so as to terminate the clinical drug effects of infused drugs at any predetermined times. I would use these types of pump when administering total intravenous anesthesia. However, while very the basic theory underlying all intravenous infusions has been dealt with in this chapter, the mathematical principles underlying the algorithms driving these computer controlled pumps, as well as their practical clinical use are subjects of more advanced theory and practice than I want to teach you at this moment."

Bob and Gerry were suddenly shocked into the real world of patient care by the stentorian voice of Sister Cybele over the intercom at a perceived sound level of 150 dB, "Doctor Gerry come to the operating theater, the next patient has arrived."

Gerry startled, spilling coffee on his trousers. "What now! Ridiculous! This is work for residents. Bob, 'She who must be obeyed' calls. The lesson is finished, as is your coffee. It's time for you to work, to function as an anesthesiologist. After all, as Zarathustra said to his disciples (9), 'One requites a teacher badly if one remains merely a student.' I'm dehydrated after this long teaching session so I need another cup of coffee." With these words Gerry poured himself another cup of coffee, and started to dither between choosing a chocolate biscuit, or a biscuit with a bright, almost poisonously fluorescent orange filling.

Bob rose, leaving Gerry alone to make the difficult choice between the two biscuits. He knew Gerry was a chocoholic, but with his sweet tooth would ultimately decide to eat both biscuits. Slowly he walked to the operating theater in some trepidation of the formidable Sister Cybele. Bob knew from working with her earlier that she was in a particularly foul humor. So it was that people passing him on his way to the operating theater thought they heard him moaning, "Why me? Why? Why?"

# 10

# A foot in the door

"Sister, how many times do I have to tell you I don't want any diathermy?" said Doctor Stanley Bigfinger in an irritated voice. "Okay, the wound is oozing slightly, but why should I cook the meat for the bacteria as well as killing it for them?" He was performing a cystectomy on a man with extensive bladder cancer, and the large and raw wound bed was bleeding from multiple sites. This did not seem to worry Bigfinger, a massive bodied, blunt mannered urologist—nicknamed "Stan the Man"—who was reputed only ever to shy back from cutting through the aorta or vena cava. Stan considered bleeding from all other abdominal blood vessels as minor oozing. His favorite form of hemostasis were the "three-P's"—Pressure, Perseverance, and if that fails, Prayer.

Bob, Gerry, and Sister Hörni looked at each other and heaved a mutual sigh. It was one of those days. All hands were needed on deck to man the pumps. Another ten bags of blood and three bags of fresh frozen plasma were ordered from the blood bank at the same time as six bags of blood and other fluids were rapidly infused into the unfortunate patient through a blood warmer. The wound kept bleeding and bleeding. Gerry went to the telephone to wheedle some units of platelet concentrate. Bob kept pumping blood and other fluids through a fluid warmer. More and more blood and fresh plasma were ordered by Gerry at the same time as he administered anesthetic drugs. Hörni organized the piles of empty blood bags, brought new bags of fluids, and kept the anesthetic chart up to date. And it kept on bleeding: three liters, five liters, and more...

Eventually the blood loss was so extreme that Gerry finally said in a firm voice, "Stan, stop operating now and apply your famous three-P's, otherwise the patient will bleed to death!" Stan stopped operating and applied his three-P's. He knew better than to disobey when Gerry used that tone of voice. Gerry continued, "We'll have to wait for more blood and platelets before you can continue. You're losing blood faster than we can replace it, and as you must have seen, the patient doesn't seem to be clotting properly any more."

"Okay Gerry," said Bigfinger, "I'll continue pressure for a few minutes, then I'll go to the coffee room until you give me the word." He filled the abdomen and pelvis with wet surgical gauze and applied pressure. Evidently the first two "P's" were all that were necessary, so after several minutes Bigfinger, his assistant, and the scrub nurse left for the coffee room.

Peace and quiet returned to the operating theater. Gerry leaned against the anesthetic machine, turned to Bob, and said, "Did you know that the decline in blood platelet concentration due to peroperative blood loss can be described with a single compartment pharmacokinetic model expressed by this simple exponential equation (1)?"

$$P = P_i \, e^{-(BL/TBV)}$$

- $P$ = actual platelet count
- $P_i$ = initial platelet count

- e = a transcendental number with the value 2.718
- BL = blood loss
- TBV = total blood volume

Bob began to get a depressing feeling that Gerry could squeeze a pharmacokinetic lesson out of just about any situation. He realized the inevitability of yet another learning moment. Just now he was tired and had little interest. He sighed inwardly as he replied, "Oh, is it relevant?"

"Very," was Gerry's succinct rejoinder.

Hörni knew from experience what to do. She simply said, "I haven't had a break yet, and the situation is stable, so if you're both going to just stand here, then I'll go and have a cup of coffee too." Having said this, she walked purposefully off in search of coffee.

"Bob, when you consider peroperative blood loss and platelet concentration, you quickly realize that the body can be viewed as a bag of blood containing a fixed number of platelets. Surgical blood loss causes loss of blood containing platelets. If the volume of lost blood is replaced at the same rate as it is lost, the concentration of platelets in the patient's blood is continually diluted by the volume replacement fluid, and the platelet concentration declines exponentially. Indeed, in the specific situation of blood volume replacement at the same rate as it is lost, platelet concentration halves with each 69.3% (about 70%) loss of total blood volume (1). I'll work out an example for this patient."

- Weight of this patient = 80 kg.
- Blood volume = 75 ml/kg (Table 3.1).
- Therefore the total blood volume of this patient = 80 x 75 = 6,000 ml.

- We know his preoperative platelet concentration was 300,000 per mm$^3$.

- We replaced his operative blood volume loss as it occurred with equivalent volumes of blood, together with fresh frozen plasma, and a plasma volume expander.

- After loss of 4,200 ml blood, which is 70% of his circulating blood volume, the platelet concentration would have been about 150,000 per mm$^3$.

- After loss of a further 4,200 ml blood, which is another 70% of his circulating blood volume, the platelet concentration would have halved yet again to about 75,000 per mm$^3$.

- This is a level at which a platelet transfusion is needed during major surgery, which is why we gave a platelet transfusion.

"But if the preoperative platelet concentration is much lower, then the volume of blood loss at which you must consider a platelet transfusion is much lower. For example, if this patient had a preoperative platelet concentration of 110,000 per mm$^3$, then a peroperative loss of 70% of the circulating blood volume, while the lost blood volume was replaced at the same rate as it was lost, would have caused the platelet concentration to drop to 55,000 per mm$^3$, and a platelet transfusion would have been needed much sooner."

"That's a useful rule-of-thumb," was Bob's reaction. "It certainly takes the guesswork out of deciding when to transfuse platelets. I like it."

Just then, the platelets, as well as more blood and fresh frozen plasma arrived. The platelets were rapidly transfused into the patient, followed by the plasma and the blood. Hörni, Bigfinger, and the rest of the operating team were recalled and recommenced the operation. Finally, after fifteen liters blood loss, the operation was finished and the patient placed on a ventilator in the intensive care unit. Stan the Man certainly knew how to keep an anesthetic team busy. "Bob, we're finished here. Now it's time for coffee," said Gerry in a firm and definite tone.

Shortly afterwards Bob and Gerry sat together in Gerry's room with steaming mugs of hot coffee in their hands. "Ah, delicious," sighed Gerry. "I can feel all the synapses in my brain just quivering with excitement in anticipation of all that caffeine. Well Bob, this is the last day of my mentorship. I think you learned some useful things during this last year. Have you any comments?"

Before Bob could answer, a loud knocking was heard on the door, which then opened slightly to admit the head of a man who peered into the room. It was Bill Pillpeddler, an English drug company representative. Bill was an unattractive, pasty-skinned man with irregular protruding yellow teeth, who appeared to live on a vitamin-free diet in a dank and sunless environment. He was also a very persistent man who never took no for an answer, and was totally unstoppable once he managed to get his foot in the door and start talking. "I hope I'm not interrupting anything Doctor Gerry," he said in a bright and irritatingly cheerful voice as he walked into the room, "but I was in the hospital visiting the pharmacist, and thought I might pop in here because I have something that will certainly interest you."

"I doubt it Bill. But who knows?" replied Gerry. "Bob pay attention. This might be interesting for you, because I know Pillpeddler's company has just introduced a new opiate on the market that is said to have some unique properties. I hadn't made an appointment with Pillpeddler because I knew he would hunt me down one day. If he wants to try and peddle this new drug, then this visit could possibly even be didactically opportune."

Bob nodded his acquiescence.

"Okay Bill, have a cup of coffee. What have you got? I've heard your company has something new."

Pillpeddler could hardly wait. He opened his case and pulled out a beautiful glossy folder filled with colorful graphs and many pictures of patients, doctors, and nurses in the exceedingly well-equipped recovery room of some hospital. Many of the patients pictured on these photographs appeared to be in some sort of drug-induced euphoric state—they were smiling, and some were even laughing. Gerry had never seen patients smiling or laughing like that in a recovery room. His experience was that patients in recovery rooms very seldom smiled—they moaned sometimes, or gritted their teeth, but they never laughed. "Here it is—our new opiate. We expect this to cause a revolution in postoperative analgesia. That's why we call it Wondorphine."

"Sounds, errr... wonderful," replied Gerry in a cautious tone.

Pillpeddler was evidently descended from a long line of irrepressible door-to-door salesmen who regarded being set-upon by dogs, or having doors painfully slamming shut in their faces, as cries of welcome and interest in their products. So he interpreted Gerry's cautious words as a manifestation of delirious enthusiasm. He happily began pulling one article reprint after the other out of his bag, each one proving Wondorphine to be better than all other opiates with which it was compared. "Okay, okay, spare me the sales talk and the articles," said Gerry. "I can work out the uses of this drug without any need to look at this mound of suspect studies. Just give me the pharmacokinetic and pharmacodynamic parameters, and I'll tell you the indications and ways to use Wondorphine."

Bill dove into his case and quickly pulled out an extensive information bulletin as well as a few articles. "I had a sneaking suspicion you might ask this question, so I took these with me. I think this is the information you want."

Gerry made a list of the parameters that interested him. "Here we are, let's have a look at what we've got. Hmmm... Interesting, I'll make a list of the relevant parameters for Wondorphine."

- MW = 420.3 g/mole.
- Moderately fat-soluble.
- pKa =7.01, and it is a base.
- $t_{1/2\alpha}$ = 10 min.
- $t_{1/2\beta}$ = 1000 min.
- $V_c$ = 0.25 l/kg.
- $V_d$ = 2 l/kg.
- Cl= 1.39 ml/kg/min= 0.0832 l/kg/hr.
- $t_{1/2}k_{e0}$ = 1.3 min.
- $EC_{50}$ (postoperative analgesia) = 1 mg/l.
- $EC_{50}$ (clinically significant respiratory depression) =10 mg/l.

Gerry studied these parameters for several seconds, and turned to Bill, "This is really a very complete data set. I'm impressed. This is unique. I've never managed to get such a complete set of parameters from a drug representative before. The national drug registration boards must be getting really finicky if you have to provide information as detailed as this. Tell me, what does your company think are the main uses for Wondorphine?"

Bob interjected, "Hang on a bit... Here you've got all the parameters, but sometimes I see that the parameter sets for anesthetic drugs are incomplete. For example, when I look at some publications I see they only give infusion rates, or clearances, or that the volume of distribution is missing, etc, etc. What do you do if you've got an inadequate set of pharmacokinetic and pharmacodynamic parameters like that?"

"There's not really much you can do about it if the parameter set really is deficient, but in some situations you can derive the values of the missing parameters from the available data. In situations where you know the clearance and infusion rate, you can calculate the plasma concentration causing a given effect by using the standard infusion equation (Chapter 9)."

$$Q = C_{ss} \times Cl$$

"Furthermore, ($\beta$, $t_{1/2\beta}$, $V_d$, and Cl are related to one another according to the equations below, which means you can easily derive one of the missing parameters from the other two."

$$\beta = 0.693 / t_{1/2\beta} = 0.693 \times V_d / Cl$$

"I see," said Bob. "That's clear enough, and even self evident when you look at it like that. Sorry about the interruption Bill, you were just about to tell us what your company expects the main uses of Wondorphine to be."

"All the studies we have done indicate that that Wondorphine is most suited as a postoperative analgesic because of its long elimination half-life. This long elimination half-life is also the reason why it is unsuited for intra-operative use, or for infusions."

"What do you think Bob?" asked Gerry.

"I agree with Bill, the long elimination half-life does appear to indicate it is unsuitable for administration by infusion. But this drug is unique as regards postoperative analgesia. It has a $t_{1/2}k_{e0} = 1.3$ minutes, which is not surprising considering the pKa = 7.01 and the fact it is a base, together with its low molecular weight. This $t_{1/2}k_{e0}$ is far lower than that of any other opiate in current use for postoperative analgesia, and means patients will have rapid pain relief after intravenous administration. Furthermore, the long elimination half-life together with an $EC_{50}$ for clinically significant respiratory depression that is ten times higher than the $EC_{50}$ for postoperative analgesia means you can select a dose that results in extremely long analgesia. I'll do an example calculation to work out a bolus dose of Wondorphine giving a period of postoperative analgesia equal in duration to its elimination half-life."

- To begin with, the $EC_{50}$ for postoperative analgesia = 1 mg/1.
- If the plasma Wondorphine concentration must remain at a level at least two times that of the $EC_{50}$ = 1 mg/l for most people to experience postoperative analgesia for a period equal to one elimination half-life, then the desired plasma Wondorphine concentration after complete drug distribution must = 2 mg/1 (see appendix for explanation).
- The volume of distribution of Wondorphine = $V_d$ = 2 l/kg.
- Plasma drug concentration after distribution without elimination = Dose/$V_d$. Accordingly, the desired Wondorphine dose = $C_{desired}$ x $V_d$ = 2 x 2 = 4 mg/kg.
- After full distribution of an intravenous 4 mg/kg bolus dose of Wondorphine, the plasma concentration will be 2 mg/1.
- And after a period equal to one elimination half-life = 1 x $t_{1/2\beta}$ = 1000 min, the plasma Wondorphine concentration will halve to 1 mg/1, which is the Wondorphine $EC_{50}$ for postoperative analgesia.
- So a Wondorphine dose of 4 mg/kg will certainly give a period of postoperative analgesia lasting 1000 minutes, which is one elimination half-life.

"Very good Bob," came the approving response from Gerry, "but I do believe you missed something."

"One moment please, I wasn't finished yet," rejoined Bob. "After all, the big question is what happens if we give this long-lasting analgesic dose as a single intravenous bolus dose to induce rapid analgesia in a patient with severe postoperative pain. Here we go again."

- Wondorphine is first present in the central compartment after a bolus dose.
- The volume of the Wondorphine central compartment = $V_c = 0.25$ l/kg.
- So the initial plasma Wondorphine concentration after an intravenous bolus of 4 mg/kg = Dose/$V_c$ = 4/0.25 = 16 mg/l.
- This initial plasma Wondorphine concentration will certainly have an analgesic effect, because it is very much higher than the $EC_{50}$ for postoperative analgesia = 1 mg/l.
- But the Wondorphine $EC_{50}$ for respiratory depression = 10 mg/l.
- This means that rapid intravenous administration of a 4 mg/kg dose of Wondorphine will quite possibly cause respiratory depression, or even apnea.
- Obviously you couldn't administer such a bolus dose of Wondorphine to an awake person without causing respiratory depression or apnea. But such a 4 mg/kg bolus dose could be administered as part of an anesthetic technique...

"Go on Bob, I like what I'm hearing," encouraged Gerry.

Bob continued, "The more I think about it, the more I realize Wondorphine is also an ideal opiate for use during anesthesia because it has a $t_{1/2}k_{e0} = 1.3$ minutes, which means it will act rapidly, and can even be used in response to acute pain. You can use a bolus dose of 4 mg/kg as an intraoperative analgesic during an anesthetic technique using controlled respiration, because then it won't matter if the patient doesn't breathe. Furthermore it has a $t_{1/2\alpha} = 10$ minutes, and distribution will essentially be finished after three to four times the distribution half-life, which is a time about equal to 30 to 40 minutes, a time period during which practically no plasma elimination will occur. Accordingly, after 30 to 40 minutes the plasma and effect compartment concentrations will have dropped to 2 mg/1, a concentration far below the $EC_{50}$ for respiratory depression, but adequate for prolonged postoperative analgesia. So, here you actually have an ideal dosage regimen for relatively short operations. This is just one example, but it does imply that with the appropriate dosage regimens, Wondorphine is a drug that can be used for both intraoperative and postoperative analgesia."

"Well reasoned Bob, but you can also use this drug in infusions too, because an infusion can also be used to administer a loading dose."

Bill looked in amazement at Bob and Gerry. In the space of a few short minutes these two anesthesiologists had worked out applications and dosages of Wondorphine that his company had only learned about by dint of several years of expensive studies in many hospitals. And they did this just by applying simple arithmetic and reasoning to known pharmacokinetic and pharmacodynamic parameters! Furthermore, they were able to work out even more potential uses by these same means! This was a totally new way of looking at drug actions for Pillpedler.

Gerry continued, "I'll work out what happens if you administer 4 mg/kg Wondorphine as an infusion."

- If you administer Wondorphine as an infusion, then it will take a time equal to at least 3 x $t_{1/2\beta}$ = 3 x 1000 minutes before your infusion achieves steady state concentrations in venous blood. This is not an option for practical anesthesia.
- But let's consider arterial drug concentrations instead of venous drug concentrations as we did before (Chapter 9).
- Average body weight of an adult = 70 kg.
- Average cardiac output of an average adult at rest = 5 1/min.
- An intravenous bolus dose = 4 mg/kg means a total dose of Wondorphine in an average adult = 4 x 70 = 280 mg.
- Wondorphine is moderately fat-soluble. So it is a reasonable assumption to say that plasma and blood Wondorphine concentrations are approximately equal.
- Desired maximum plasma Wondorphine concentration = 2 mg/1.
- If one assumes insignificant venous recirculation, then the [arterial drug concentration] = [drug infusion rate] / [cardiac output].
- Accordingly the desired Wondorphine infusion rate = [desired arterial concentration] x [cardiac output] = 2 x 5 = 10 mg/min.
- Therefore the number of minutes over which the 280 mg dose of Wondorphine must be administered so that the infusion rate is never more than 10 mg/min = 280/10 = 28 minutes.
- So if Wondorphine is infused at a rate of 10 mg/min to an average 70 kg adult for about 30 minutes, then that person will have a blood Wondorphine concentration of not much more than 2 mg/1. Yet at the same time that person will receive a loading dose of 4 mg/kg without develop-

ing any significant respiratory depression. In other words, such an infusion can be administered intraoperatively, as well as postoperatively.

- Furthermore, patients will experience rapid analgesia because of the short $t_{1/2}k_{e0}$ of Wondorphine.

Bill and Bob looked at each other. Gerry could see they were impressed. He continued, "So as you see, you can use Wondorphine as a useful anesthetic analgesic which has the added advantage of causing long lasting postoperative analgesia. Its short $t_{1/2}k_{e0}$ means it is a very useful drug to administer in reaction to pain. There is one more aspect to the intraoperative use of this drug. Most operations last less than three hours, which is a time very much shorter than the elimination half-life of Wondorphine. Even though Wondorphine has a useful difference between the $EC_{50}$ for clinically significant respiratory depression and the $EC_{50}$ for postoperative analgesia, if you administer too much during an operation, regardless of whether you do this by intermittent bolus dosages, or by an infusion—too high a total intraoperative dose will cause extremely long-lasting postoperative respiratory depression. This will certainly limit the maximum usable intraoperative dosage. So what is the maximum usable intraoperative Wondorphine dosage above which long-lasting postoperative respiratory depression, or apnea will be likely? Let's calculate this maximum intraoperative dose of Wondorphine."

- The Wondorphine $EC_{50}$ for clinically significant respiratory depression = 10 mg/1. But this is an average, which means that 50% of people will develop respiratory depression at lower plasma Wondorphine concentrations. So let us assume for the sake of this example, that no-one experiences clinically significant respiratory depression at plasma Wondorphine concentrations below 7 mg/1.

- This means that before an operation ends, full distribution must have occurred, so that the maximum plasma concentration of Wondorphine is no higher than 7 mg/1 at the end of the operation.
- The distribution volume of Wondorphine = $V_d$ = 2 l/kg.
- Accordingly, the intraoperative dose of Wondorphine required to produce a plasma concentration of 7 mg/1 after full distribution has occurred = Dose x $V_d$ = 7 x 2 = 14 mg/kg.
- Accordingly the maximum intraoperative dose of Wondorphine is 14 mg/kg. This dose of Wondorphine can be administered by intermittent bolus, or as an infusion.

Gerry continued. "It's always possible that such a maximum 14 mg/kg dose is inadequate to provide sufficient analgesia for some operations. In such cases, you can always be practical and administer extra analgesia with a Remifentanil infusion. Turn off the Remifentanil at the end of the operation, and you have the residual long-lasting analgesia of Wondorphine—another way of using Wondorphine. You can go on and on in this way to devise many different ways to use Wondorphine." Gerry turned to Bob, and asked, "Can you think of anything you or I might have missed?"

Bob shook his head, "No, nothing at all."

Gerry continued, "Well Bill, your company calls it Wondorphine—and they're right—it is a Wondorphine, because if these parameters on which we based our predictions are reasonably accurate, then it can be used in many ways."

Bill was really impressed. "You've predicted most of our clinical experimental results, and provided a few new suggestions I'm sure our clinical research department will want to follow up on. I have to go to another appointment now, but I'll leave you these folders and articles. In addition, I'm going to speak to my bosses about what you just did. Perhaps we could arrange something with you in the future? I'll get back to you soon on the results of my talk." So it was that a happy and much wiser Pillpedler departed for his next appointment.

"So Bob, what a lucky coincidence that Pillpeddler came just at that moment. His visit showed me you really have mastered the essence of pharmacokinetic and pharmacodynamic reasoning." As Gerry spoke with Bob, they walked to the door of Gerry's room. It was also time for Bob to depart. Gerry spoke a few words of farewell, "Well Bob, I do believe you've learnt some useful things during your stay here. I even believe some of these things will help you throughout your future promising career as an anesthesiologist.

I'm always minded at the end of each mentorship to give a slightly paraphrased piece of advice given long ago by Lord Krishna to Prince Arjuna."

*By humble heed of those who see the Truth and teach it. Knowing Truth, thy heart no more will ache with the terror of unknowing, for the Truth shall show all things subdued to thee,...(2)*

This quotation, together with the last demonstration of the power of physiological, pharmacokinetic, pharmacodynamic reasoning had a startlingly sudden and profound effect on Bob. His face changed, transfigured by an expression of total awe. He stood still, paralyzed by the overwhelming intensity of his emotions. Tears welled from his eyes, rolling down his cheeks. His widened pupils stared at something unseen, but clearly unspeakably wonderful. All he had learned finally culminated in an ecstatic state—a profound anesthesiological, physiological, pharmacokinetic, and pharmacodynamic epiphany. He managed to croak, "Thank you, thank you for teaching me these things," as he wrung

Gerry's hands before stumbling out of the room, a transformed and better man. Sister Hörni entered as he left. She saw the condition of Doctor Bob. She understood the cause of his transfiguration, knew what he was experiencing, and saw that it was good. Another young doctor had learned understanding of the basic truths of anesthesia.

"Shall we go home?" she asked Gerry.

"Yes, let's. It's late, the dogs must be getting lonely."

# Appendix

## Kinetic and Dynamic Parameters

### A very important note...

Pharmacokinetic and pharmacodynamic data are listed throughout this book as well as in this appendix. It cannot be emphasized enough that these data are averages, a fact applying to all biological parameters. For example, look at the tables in this appendix. The average plasma concentration of Propofol causing hypnosis is 2 mg/1. But you cannot say no one will fall asleep at a plasma Propofol concentration of 1.99999 mg/1, while everyone will suddenly fall asleep at a concentration of 2 mg/1 or higher. An average plasma hypnotic concentration of 2 mg/1 means that 50% of people will fall asleep at plasma Propofol concentrations above this level, while 50% will fall asleep at lower plasma Propofol concentrations. To think otherwise is a bit like believing that women suddenly develop hot flushes and other manifestations of the menopause only on the exact day of their 50th birthday (the average age of menopause): that people only die on the exact day of their 76th birthday (the average lifespan in some countries): that men are only exactly 175 cm (5 feet 9 inches) tall, and that women are only exactly 160 cm (5 feet 3 inches) tall (average heights of men and women in some populations). Everyone knows such beliefs are ridiculous, knowing full well these things are only averages that also vary according to the population being considered, e.g. Scandinavians are much taller than Chinese people, Asians often have lactose intolerance, Africans have dark brown eyes, etc, etc. The same applies to all pharmacokinetic, pharmacodynamic, and physiological data, because values for these parameters give an indication of the average levels of these parameters within a set population. This does not mean these parameters are worthless fantasies of no clinical value—it simply means they should be interpreted in the same way as we instinctively interpret the other averages confronting us each day of our lives.

## Kinetic model

The data listed in these tables are for a two-compartment pharmacokinetic model. A two-compartment model provides a reasonably accurate, clinically relevant description of anesthetic drug kinetics after intravenous bolus injection, as well as during relatively short infusions (1). Furthermore, the two-compartment model is an invaluable model for the purposes of acquiring clinical insights and performing clinically relevant calculations.

## Pharmacokinetic variables

The meanings of pharmacokinetic variables such as $t_{1/2\alpha}$, $\alpha$, $t_{1/2\beta}$, $\beta$, $V_\beta$, $V_d$, $t_{1/2}k_{e0}$, and Cl have been explained in the text of Chapter 3. Readers should note that these tables use the units "1/h/kg" for clearance instead of the more usual "ml/min/kg". This is done for two reasons: drug concentrations at which effects occur are given as mg/1, as well as to simplify calculation of drug infusion rates.

## EC$_{50}$

EC$_{50}$ is the effective steady state plasma concentration of a drug sufficient to induce a given pharmacological effect in 50% of people. Drug concentrations 2-3 times the $EC_{50}$ are usually required to produce that same effect in more than 90% of persons.

## $EC_{50}$ for hypnosis

These are the effective steady state plasma concentrations of hypnotic drugs capable of inducing hypnosis with loss of the eyelid reflex in 50% of people. Note that the plasma concentration of a drug required to induce only hypnosis is less than the concentration required to induce hypnosis with loss of eyelid or pain reflexes (see Table 9.1).

## $EC_{90}$ for muscle relaxation

Non-depolarizing muscle relaxant effect is usually quantified by measuring the contraction force of an adductor pollicis longus muscle in response to supramaximal electrical stimulation of the ulnar nerve innervating it. The values for $EC_{90}$ are the steady state plasma effective concentrations of muscle relaxants causing 90% twitch height depression in 50% of people. The $EC_{90}$ is a concentration of muscle relaxant sufficient to permit intra-abdominal surgery, and is a concentration at which it is possible to measure one to two twitches in response to a train-of-four stimulation.

## $EC_{50}$ for postoperative analgesia

These are the effective minimum steady state plasma concentrations of opiates capable of inducing effective postoperative analgesia in 50% of awake and spontaneously breathing patients. This level is chosen simply because intraoperative opiate demands are too diverse for a list to make any sense. Higher plasma opiate concentrations are usually required for surgery to be possible.

## EC$_{50}$ for tachycardia

These are the effective minimum steady state plasma concentrations of anticholinergic drugs capable of inducing a tachycardia in 50% of people.

## EC$_{50}$ for inotropic effect

These are the effective minimum steady state plasma concentrations of inotropic drugs required to exert an inotropic effect in 50% of people for each of any one of this diverse group of drugs.

## Molecular weight

Molecular weight is not an average, but an absolute physicochemical measurement. The larger the molecular weight of a molecule, the slower it diffuses out of capillaries. This is one of the reasons why the $t_{1/2}k_{e0}$ of a drug with a larger molecular weight is longer than that of a drug with a smaller molecular weight (also see end of Chapter 3).

## pKa

The pKa of a drug is the pH at which 50% of that drug exists in the ionized form. Just as with molecular weight, the pKa is also an absolute physico-chemical measurement.

The addition of an "a" to the listed pKa value means that the drug is an acid, while the addition of a "b" means that the drug is a base. This is not a usual convention, but I have done it for the sake of clarity to explain the behavior of some drugs. Here are some examples showing the use of the pKa (also see the end of Chapter 3).

*Appendix*

- Alfentanil is a molecule with a pKa = 6.1. It is also a base. A base is always less ionized at higher pH levels, and more ionized at lower pH levels. At a pH = 6.1, about 50% of all the Alfentanil molecules are ionized—and Alfentanil is a base—so at blood pH = 7.4, less than 50% of the Alfentanil in blood is ionized. Unionized molecules diffuse more rapidly than ionized molecules, and this also partly explains why the $t_{1/2}k_{e0}$ of Alfentanil is so short. This is quite different for Sufentanil whose pKa = 8.1, which means that most Sufentanil is ionized at blood pH. Ionized molecules attract a cloud of other oppositely charged molecules around them. This effectively enlarges their molecular diameters, and slows their speeds of diffusion. This partly explains the longer $t_{1/2}k_{e0}$ of a drug such as Sufentanil.

- Muscle relaxants have a high pKa and are also bases. This means that muscle relaxant molecules are highly ionized in blood with a pH = 7.4. This also partly explains the longer $t_{1/2}k_{e0}$ values of non-depolarizing muscle relaxant drugs.

## INDUCTION AGENTS

| DRUG | MW (g/mole) | pKa | $t_{1/2\alpha}$ (min) | $t_{1/2\beta}$ (min) | $V_c$ (l/kg) | $V_d$ (l/kg) | Cl (l/kg/h) | $EC_{50}$ (hypnosis) (mg/l) | $t_{1/2}k_{e0}$ (min) |
|---|---|---|---|---|---|---|---|---|---|
| Thiopental | 264.33 | 7.6a | 3.3[2] | 781 | 0.128 | 3.5 | 0.19 | 10 | 1.2 |
| Methohexital | 284.3 | 7.9a | 5.6[3] | 234 | 0.38 | 3.7 | 0.65 | 3.4 | ? |
| Hexobarbital | 236.26 | | 23.4[4] | 299 | 0.54 | 1.4 | 0.2 | 10 | ? |
| Ketamine | 237.74 | 7.5b | 11[5] | 151 | 0.86 | 4 | 1.1 | 1 | ? |
| Etomidate | 244.28 | 4.24b | 2.6[6] | 57 | 0.3 | 2.2 | 1.39 | 0.21 | 1.6 |
| Propofol | 178.3 | 11.1b | 2.5[7] | 55 | 0.63 | 4.7 | 3.55 | 2 | 2.9 |

## ANTICHOLINERGICS

| DRUG | MW (g/mole) | pKa | $t_{1/2\alpha}$ (min) | $t_{1/2\beta}$ (min) | $V_c$ (l/kg) | $V_d$ (l/kg) | Cl (l/kg/h) | $EC_{50}$ (tachycardia) (mg/l) | $t_{1/2}k_{e0}$ (min) |
|---|---|---|---|---|---|---|---|---|---|
| Atropine | 289.38 | 9.8b | 1.7[8] | 180 | 0.09 | 1.6 | 0.41 | 0.03 | ? |
| Scopolamine | 303.35 | | 5.4[8] | 114 | 0.2 | 1.1 | 0.81 | 0.03 | ? |

## ANTICHOLINESTERASES

| DRUG | MW (g/mole) | pKa | $t_{1/2\alpha}$ (min) | $t_{1/2\beta}$ (min) | $V_c$ (l/kg) | $V_d$ (l/kg) | Cl (l/kg/h) | $EC_{50}$ (mg/l) | $t_{1/2}k_{e0}$ (min) |
|---|---|---|---|---|---|---|---|---|---|
| Neostigmine | 334.39 | | 3.4[9] | 77 | 0.22 | 1.02 | 0.55 | ? | ? |
| Edrophonium | 246.15 | | 7.2[9] | 110 | 0.32 | 1.53 | 0.58 | ? | ? |
| Pyridostigmine | 261.14 | | 6.8[10] | 112 | 0.3 | 1.4 | 0.52 | ? | ? |

## MUSCLE RELAXANTS

| DRUG | MW (g/mole) | pKa | $t_{1/2\alpha}$ (min) | $t_{1/2\beta}$ (min) | $V_c$ (l/kg) | $V_d$ (l/kg) | Cl (l/kg/h) | $EC_{90}$ (surgical relaxation) (mg/l) | $t_{1/2}k_{e0}$ (min) |
|---|---|---|---|---|---|---|---|---|---|
| Gallamine | 891.56 | >13b | 6.7[11] | 144 | 0.1 | 0.23 | 0.065 | 7.2 | ? |
| Tubocurarine | 771.84 | 8.6b | 6.2[12] | 119 | 0.1 | 0.39 | 0.135 | 0.63 | 4.7 |
| Alcuronium | 737.8 | | 13.8[13] | 199 | 0.13 | 0.4 | 0.083 | 0.66 | ? |
| Pancuronium | 732.7 | >13b | 10.7[14] | 114 | 0.12 | 0.3 | 0.11 | 0.27 | 3.3 |
| Vecuronium | 637.75 | | 7.5[15] | 53 | 0.09 | 0.4 | 0.32 | 0.15 | 3.7 |
| Rocuronium | 609.7 | | 14.8[16] | 97.2 | 0.038 | 0.21 | 0.22 | 2 | 4.3 |
| Atracurium | 1243.51 | | 2[17] | 21 | 0.07 | 0.2 | 0.32 | 1.13 | 5.9 |
| Mivacurium | 1100.18 | | ?[18] | 2 | ? | 0.2 | 4.2 | 0.1 | 6.9 |
| Sugammadex | 2002 | | ?[42] | 136 | 0.033 | 0.11 | 0.063 | NR | ? |

## OPIATES

| DRUG | MW (g/mole) | pKa | $t_{1/2\alpha}$ (min) | $t_{1/2\beta}$ (min) | $V_c$ (l/kg) | $V_d$ (l/kg) | Cl (l/kg/h) | EC$_{50}$ (postop. analgesia) (mg/l) | $t_{1/2}k_{e0}$ (min) |
|---|---|---|---|---|---|---|---|---|---|
| Morphine | 285.33 | 7.93b | 4.4[19] | 111 | 1.01 | 5.4 | 2.01 | 0.015 | 20 |
| Methadone | 345.9 | 9.26b | 6.1[20] | 2100 | 1.1 | 8.2 | 0.016 | 0.03 | ? |
| Meperidine | 247.34 | 8.5b | 4.1[21] | 192 | 0.63 | 3.3 | 0.72 | 0.46 | ? |
| Pentazocine | 285.44 | 9.16b | ?[22] | 204 | ? | 5.6 | 1.2 | 0.1 | ? |
| Buprenorphine | 504.1 | 8.51b | 2.1[23] | 140 | 0.132 | 2.69 | 0.8 | 0.001 | ? |
| Piritramide | 416.5 | | 4[24] | 480 | 0.7 | 4.7 | 0.47 | 0.012 | 16.8 |
| Phenoperidine | 403.9 | 8.01b | 2.2[25] | 193 | 0.9 | 6.13 | 1.32 | 0.005 | ? |
| Fentanyl | 528.61 | 8.4b | 9[26] | 263 | 0.77 | 3.81 | 0.65 | 0.001 | 6.4 |
| Alfentanil | 471 | 6.5b | 3.8[27] | 67 | 0.17 | 0.54 | 0.33 | 0.1 | 1.1 |
| Sufentanil | 578.69 | 8.01b | 1.4[28] | 164 | 0.16 | 2.9 | 0.76 | 0.0001 | 5.8 |
| Remifentanil | 412.92 | 7.07b | ?[29] | 9.52 | ? | 0.35 | 2.5 | 0.005 | 1.3 |

**ANTAGONISTS & ANALEPTICS**

| DRUG | MW (g/mole) | pKa | $t_{1/2\alpha}$ (min) | $t_{1/2\beta}$ (min) | $V_c$ (l/kg) | $V_d$ (l/kg) | Cl (l/kg/h) | $EC_{50}$ (mg/l) | $t_{1/2}k_{e0}$ (min) |
|---|---|---|---|---|---|---|---|---|---|
| Naloxone | 327.37 | 7.82b | 1.8[30] | 19 | 0.81 | 2.4 | 5.3 | ? | ? |
| Doxapram | 378.5 | | 5.3[31] | 54 | 0.44 | 3.2 | 0.36 | 3 | ? |
| Physostigmine | 275.34 | | 2.3[32] | 22 | ? | 0.6 | 1.2 | 0.004 | ? |
| Flumazanil | 303.3 | | ?[33] | 58 | ? | 0.82 | 0.6 | 0.02 | ? |

**INOTROPICS**

| DRUG | MW (g/mole) | pKa | $t_{1/2\alpha}$ (min) | $t_{1/2\beta}$ (min) | $V_c$ (l/kg) | $V_d$ (l/kg) | Cl (l/kg/h) | $EC_{50}$ (mg/l) | $t_{1/2}k_{e0}$ (min) |
|---|---|---|---|---|---|---|---|---|---|
| Epinephrine | 183.2 | | 3.1[34,35] | 10.9 | ? | 1.89 | 7.2 | 0.0001 | ? |
| Norepinephrine | 205.2 | | 2[36] | 34 | ? | 1.96 | 2.4 | 0.0018 | ? |
| Isoprenaline | 247.72 | | 3[37] | 240 | ? | ? | ? | ? | ? |
| Ephedrine | 165.24 | | ?[38] | 405 | ? | 3.18 | 0.36 | ? | ? |
| Dopamine | 153 | | 0.9[39] | 9.2 | ? | 0.89 | 4.32 | 0.07 | ? |
| Dobutamine | 337.84 | | ?[40] | 2.37 | ? | 0.2 | 3.6 | 0.042 | ? |
| Digoxin | 781 | | ?[41] | 41.2 hr | ? | 14.5 | 0.258 | >0.0008 | ? |

# References

## Chapter 1

Clutter WE, et al. (1980) Adrenaline plasma clearance rates and physiologic thresholds for metabolic and hemodynamic actions in man. *The Journal of Clinical Investigation*, 66: 94-101.

Fitzgerald GA, et al. (1980) Circulating adrenaline and blood pressure: the metabolic effects and kinetics of infused adrenaline in man. *European Journal of Clinical Investigation*, 10: 401-406.

Grotte G, (1956), Passage of dextran molecules across the blood-lymph barrier. *Acta Chirurgica Scandinavica*, supplement 211: 5-84.

Altman PL, et al (eds.), (1959), *Handbook of Circulation*, pub. W.B. Saunders, U.S.A., 1959, Library of Congress No. 59-15183.

## Chapter 2

*1. Koran*, (1990), Dawood NJ, (translator)Published by Penguin Books, England. Sura 39, verse 42.

2. Slutsky R, et al, (1982) Pulmonary blood volume. Correlation of radionucleotide and dye-dilution estimates. *Investigative Radiology*, 17: 233-240.

3. Lewis ML, et al, (1970), Determinants of pulmonary blood volume. *The Journal of Clinical Investigation*, 49: 170-182.

4. Hudson RJ, et al, (1983), A model for studying depth of Anesthesia and acute tolerance to Thiopentone. *Anesthesiology*, 59: 301-308.

5. Kissin I, et al, (1983), Inotropic and anesthetic potencies of etomidate and Thiopentone in dogs. *Anesthesia & Analgesia*, 62: 961-965.

6. Lauven PM, et al, (1985), Venous threshold concentrations o methohexitone. *Anesthesiology*, 63: A368.

7. Schüttler J, et al, (1985), Infusion strategies to investigate the pharmacokinetics and pharmacodynamics of hypnotic drugs: etomidate as an example. *European Journal of Anaesthesiology*, 2: 133-142.

8. Barr J, et al, (1999), Propofol dosing regimens for ICU sedation based upon an integrated pharmacokinetic-pharmacodynamic model. *Anesthesiology*, 95: 324-333.

9. Goodchild CS, Serrao JM, (1989), Cardiovascular effects of propofol in the anaesthetized dog. *British Journal of Anaesthesia*, 63: 87-92.

10. Bennetts FE, (1995), Thiopentone anaesthesia at Pearl Harbor. *British Journal of Anaesthesia*, 75, 366-368.
11. Altman PL, et al (eds.), (1959), *Handbook of Circulation*, pub. W.B. Saunders, U.S.A., 1959, Library of Congress No. 59-15183, pages 115-125.
12. Shafer SL, (2004), Shock Values. *Anesthesiology*, 101: 567-568
13. Upton RN, et al, (1999), Cardiac Output is a Determinant of the Initial Concentrations of Propofol After Short-Infusion Administration. *Anesthesia & Analgesia*, 89, 545-552.
14. Rossen R, et al, (1943), Acute arrest of cerebral circulation in man. *Archives of Neurology & Psychiatry*, 50: 510-528.
15. Boothby WM, (1954), *Respiratory Physiology in Aviation*. Published by the Air University, USAF School of Aviation

# Chapter 4

1. Duvaldestin P, et al, (1982), Pharmacokinetics of pancuronium in man: a linear system. *European Journal of Clinical Pharmacology*, 23: 369-72.
2. Buzello W, (1975), The metabolism of pancuronium in man. *Der Anaesthesist*, 24:13-18.
3. Donati F, Bevan DR, (1985), Antagonism of phase II succinylcholine block by neostigmine. *Anesthesia & Analgesia*, 64: 773-776.
4. Welliver M, et al, (2008), Discovery, development, and clinical applicationof sugammadex sodium, a selective relaxant binding agent. *Drug Design, Development and Therapy*, 2: 49-59
5. Staals LM, et al, (2008), Multicentre, parallel-group, comparative trial evaluating the efficacy and safety of sugammadex in patients with end-stage renal failure or normal renal function. *British Journal of Anaesthesia*, 101: 492-297.

# Chapter 5

1. *The Holy Bible*, King James Version, Ecclesiastes, chapter 12, verse 12.

# Chapter 6

1. *The Holy Bible*, King James Version, Genesis, chapter 11, verses 26-31.
2. Kazama T, et al, (2001), Relation between initial blood distribution volume and propofol induction dose requirement. *Anesthesiology*, 94: 205-210.

# References

3. Messerli FH, (1982), Cardiovascular effects of obesity and hypertension. *Lancet*, 1: 1165-1168.
4. Simone G de, et al, (1997), Stroke Volume and Cardiac Output in Normotensive Children and Adults. Assessment of Relations With Body Size and Impact of Overweight. *Circulation*, 95: 1837-1843.
5. Tarquin C, et al, (2001), Relations of Stroke Volume and Cardiac Output to Body Composition. The Strong Heart Study. *Circulation*, 103: 820-825.
6. Danias PG, et al, (2003), Cardiac structure and function in the obese: a cardiovascular magnetic resonance imaging study. *Journal of Cardiovascular Magnetic Resonance*, 5: 431-438.
7. Upton RN, et al, (1999), Cardiac Output is a Determinant of the Initial Concentrations of Propofol After Short-Infusion Administration. *Anesthesia & Analgesia*, 89: 545-552.
8. Henthorn TK, et al, (1992), The relationship between alfentanil distribution kinetics and cardiac output. *Clinical Pharmacology & Therapeutics*, 52: 190-196.
9. Wada DR, et al, (1997), Computer simulation of the effects of alterations in blood flows and body composition on thiopental pharmacokinetics in humans. *Anesthesiology*, 87: 884-899.
10. Ledgerwood AM, et al, (1992), The influence of an Anesthetic regimen on patient care, outcome, and hospital charges. *The American Surgeon*, 58: 527-533.
11. Woerlee GM, (2003), *Mortal Minds—A Biology of the Soul and the Dying Experience*, published by de Tijdstroom, The Netherlands, ISBN 905898057X, Chapter 16. (Also published under the title, *Mortal Minds— A Biology of the Near Death Experience*, published by Prometheus Books, USA, 2005, Chapter 16.)
12. Comroe JH, Botelho SAB, (1947), The unreliability of cyanosis in the recognition of arterial hypoxemia. *The American Journal of the Medical Sciences*, 214: 1 -6.

# Chapter 7

1. Ilett KF, (1997), Drug distribution in human milk. *Australian Prescriber*, 20: 35-40.
2. Sievers E, et al, (2002), Feeding patterns in breast-fed and formula-fed infants. *Annals of Nutrition and Metabolism*, 46: 243-248.
3. Wittels B, et al, (1997), Postcesarean analgesia with both epidural morphine and intravenous patient-controlled analgesia: neurobe-havioural outcome-samong nursing neonates. *Anesthesia & Analgesia*, 85: 600-606.

4. Payne JP, (1962), Apnoeic oxygenation in anaesthetised man. *Acta Anaesthesiologica Scandinavica*, 6: 129-142.
5. Eger EI, Severinghaus JW, (1961), The rate of rise of PaCO2 in the apneic anesthetized patient. *Anesthesiology*, 22: 419-425.
6. Frumin MJ, et al, (1959), Apneic oxygenation in man. *Anesthesiology*, 20: 789-798.
7. Refsum HE, (1963), Relationship between state of consciousness and arterial hypoxaemia in patients with pulmonary insufficiency, breathing air. *Clinical Science*, 25: 361-367.
8. Kety SS, Schmidt CF, (1946), The effects of active and passive hyperventilation on cerebral blood flow, cerebral oxygen consumption, cardiac output, and blood pressure of normal young men. *Journal of Clinical Investigation*, 25:107-119.
9. Alexander SC, et al, (1968), Cerebral carbohydrate metabolism of man during respiratory and metabolic alkalosis. *Journal of Applied Physiology*, 24: 66-72.
10. Wollman H, et al, (1965), Cerebral circulation during anesthesia and hyperventilation in man. *Anesthesiology*, 26: 329-334.
11. Wollman H, et al, (1968), Effects of extremes of respiratory and metabolic alkalosis on cerebral blood flow in man. *Journal of Applied Physiology*, 24: 60-65.
12. Stoddart JC, (1967), Electroencephalographic activity during voluntary controlled alveolar hyperventilation. *British Journal of Anaesthesia*, 39: 2-10.
13. Eisele JH, et al, (1967), Narcotic properties of carbon dioxide in the dog. *Anesthesiology*, 28: 856-865.
14. Frumin MJ, et al, (1959), Apneic oxygenation in man. *Anesthesiology*, 20: 789-798.

# Chapter 8

1. *Sixty Upanishads of the Veda*, translated into German by P. Deussen, and into English from German by V.M. Bedekar and G.B. Palsule, published by Motilal Banarsidass Publishers Pty Ltd, India, 1990, ISBN 81-208-0431-7, page 494.

# Chapter 9

1. Barr J, et al, (1999), Propofol dosing regimens for ICU sedation based upon an integrated pharmacokinetic-pharmacodynamic model. *Anesthesiology*, 95: 324-333.
2. White M, et al, (1999) Effect-site modelling of Propofol using auditory evoked potentials. *British Journal of Anaesthesia*, 82: 333-339.
3. Lim TA, (2003), A novel method of deriving the effect compartment equilibrium rate constant for Propofol. *British Journal of Anaesthesia*, 91: 730-732.
4. Levitt DG, (2004), Physiologically based pharmacokinetic modelling of arterial—antecubital vein concentration difference. *BMC Clinical Pharmacology*, 4: 2 (This article is available from: www.biomedcentral.eom/1472-6904/4/2).
5. Barratt RL, et al, (1984), Kinetics of thiopentone in relation to the site of sampling. *British Journal of Anaesthesia*, 56: 1385-1391.
6. Tuk B, et al, (1997), The impact of arteriovenous concentration differences on pharmacodynamic parameter estimates. *Journal of Pharmacokineics and Biopharmaceutics*, 25: 39-62.
7. Peacock JE, et al, (1995), Arterial and jugular venous bulb blood propofol concentrations during induction of anesthesia. *Anesthesia & Analgesia*, 80: 1002-1006.
8. He YL, et al, (2000), Pulmonary disposition of propofol in surgical patients. *Anesthesiology*, 93: 986-991.
9. Nietzsche F, *Thus Spoke Zarathustra*, the Thomas Common translation, part 1, chapter 22, *The Bestowing of Virtue*, part 3.

# Chapter 10

1. Miller RD, et al, (1971) Coagulation defects associated with massive blood transfusions. *Annals of Surgery*, 174: 794-801.
2. Arnold E, (translator), (1885), *The Bhagavad Gita*, Theosophical University Press Electronic Edition, ISBN 1-55700-155-3, chapter 4, stanzas 34-35.

# Appendix

1. Kanto J, Gepts E, (1989), Pharmacokinetic implications for the clinical use of propofol. *Clinical Pharmacokinetics*, 17: 308-326.
2. Christensen JH, et al, (1982), Pharmacokinetics and pharmacodynamics of thiopentone. A comparison between young and elderly patients. *Anaesthesia*, 37: 399-404.

3. Hudson RJ, et al, (1983), Pharmacokinetics of methohexital and thiopental in surgical patients. *Anesthesiology*, 59: 215-219.

4. Richter E, et al, (1980), Disposition of hexobarbital in intra- and extrahepatic cholestasis in man and the influence of drug metabolism inducing agents. *European Journal of Clinical Pharmacology*, 17: 197-202.

5. Wieber J, et al, (1975), Pharmacokinetics of ketamine in man. *Der Anaesthesist*, 24: 260-263.

6. Schüttler J, et al, (1980), Pharmakokinetische Untersuchungen uber Etomidat beim Menschen. *Der Anaesthesist*, 29: 658-661.

7. Adam HK, et al, (1983), Pharmacokinetic evaluation of ICI 35868 in man. *British Journal of Anaesthesia*, 55: 97-102.

8. Calculated on the basis of the kinetic data and the dose-effect relationship in the article: Gravenstein JS, et al, (1964), Effects of atropine and scopolamine on the cardiovascular system in man. *Anesthesiology*, 25: 123-130.

9. Morris RB, et al, (1981), Pharmacokinetics of edrophonium and neostigmine when antagonizing d-tubocurarine neuromuscular blockade in man. *Anesthesiology*, 54: 399-402.

10. Cronnelly, R., et al. (1980), Pyridostigmine kinetics with and without renal function. *Clinical Pharmacology & Therapeutics*, 28: 78-81.

11. Ramzan, M.I., et al. (1980), Pharmacokinetic studies in man with gallamine triethiodide. I .Single and multiple clinical doses. *European Journal of Clinical Pharmacology*, 17: 135-143.

12. Stanski DR, et al, (1979), Pharmacokinetics: and pharmacody-namics of d-tubocurarine during nitrous oxide-narcotic and halothane anesthesia in man. *Anesthesiology*, 51: 235-241.

13. Walker J, et al, (1988), Clinical pharmacokinetics of alcuronium in man. *European Journal of Clinical Pharmacology*, 17: 449-457.

14. Duvaldestein P, et al, (1978), Pancuronium pharmacokinetics in patients with liver cirrhosis. *British Journal of Anaesthesia*, 50: 1131-1135.

15. Lynam DP, et al, (1988), The pharmacodynamics and pharmacokinetics of vecuronium in patients anesthetized with isoflurane with normal renal function or with renal failure. *Anesthesiology*, 69: 227-231.

16. McCoy EP, et al (1996), Pharmacokinetics of rocuronium after bolus and continuous infusion during halothane anaesthesia. *British Journal of Anaesthesia*, 76: 29-33.

17. Ward S, Neill EAM, (1983), Pharmacokinetics of atracurium in acute hepatic failure (with acute renal failure). *British Journal of Anaesthesia*, 55:1169-1172.

18. Mivacurium pharmacokinetics. www.rxlist.com/cgi/generic3/miva-cur cp.htm

# References

19. Mazoit J-X, et al, (1987), Pharmacokinetics of unchanged morphine in normal and cirrhotic subjects. *Anesthesiology*, 66: 293-298.
20. Gourlay GK, et al, (1982), Pharmacokinetics and pharmacodynamics of methadone during the perioperative period. *Anesthesiology*, 57: 458-467.
21. Mather LE, et al, (1974), Meperidine kinetics in man. Intravenous injection in surgical patients and volunteers. *Clinical Pharmacology & Therapeutics*, 17: 21-30.
22. Ehrnebo M, et al, (1977), Bioavailability and first-pass metabolism of pentazocine in man. Clinical Pharmacology & Therapeutics, 22: 888-892.
23. Bullingham RES, et al, (1980), Buprenorphine kinetics. *Clinical Pharmacology & Therapeutics*, 28: 667-672.
24. Kietzmann D, et al, (1996), Pharmacokinetics of piritramide after an intravenous bolus in surgical patients. *Acta Anaesthesiologica Scandinavica*, 40: 898-903.
25. Fischler M, et al, (1985), Pharmacokinetics of phenoperidine in anaesthetized patients undergoing general surgery. *British Journal of Anaesthesia*, 57: 872-876.
26. Haberer JP, et al, (1982), Fentanyl pharmacokinetics in anaesthetized patients with cirrhosis. *British Journal of Anaesthesia*, 54: 1267-1269.
27. Schüttler J, Stoekel H, (1982), Alfentanil (R39209) ein neues kurzwerkendes Opioid. Pharmakokinetik und eerste klinische Erfahrungen. *Der Anaesthesist*, 31: 10-14.
28. Bovill JG, et al, (1984), The pharmacokinetics of sufentanil in surgical patients. *Anesthesiology*, 61: 502-506.
29. Duthie DJR, (1998), Remifentanil and Tramadol. *British Journal of Anaesthesia*, 81: 51-57.
30. Goldfrank L, et al, (1986), A dosing nomogram for continuous infusion of intravenous naloxone. *Annals of Emergency Medicine*, 15: 566-570.
31. Clements JA, et al, (1979), The disposition of intravenous doxapram in man. *European Journal of Clinical Pharmacology*, 16: 411-416.
32. Hartvig P, et al, (1986), Pharmacokinetics of physostigmine after intravenous, intramuscular and subcutaneous administration in surgical patients. *Acta Anaesthesiologica Scandinavica*, 30: 177-182.
33. Klotz U, et al, (1984), Pharmacokinetics of the selective benzodiazepine antagonist Ro 15-1788 in man. *European Journal of Clinical Pharmacology*, 27:,115-117.
34. Fitzgerald GA, et al, (1980) Circulating adrenaline and blood pressure: the metabolic effects and kinetics of infused adrenaline in man. *European Journal of Clinical Investigation*, 10: 401-406.

35. Clutter WE, et al, (1980), Adrenaline plasma clearance rates and physiologic thresholds for metabolic and hemodynamic actions in man. *The Journal of Clinical Investigation*, 66: 94-101.
36. Esler M, et al, (1981), Effect of norepinephrine uptake blockers on norepinephrine kinetics. *Clinical Pharmacology & Therapeutics*, 29: 12-20.
37. Kadar, D, et al, (1974), Isoproteranol metabolism in children after intravenous administration. *Clinical Pharmacology & Therapeutics*, 16: 789-795.
38. Pickup ME, et al, (1976), The pharmacokinetics of ephedrine after oral dosage in asthmatics receiving acute and chronic treatment. *British Journal of Clinical Pharmacology*, 3: 123-134.
39. Jarnberg PO, et al., (1981) Dopamine infusion in man. Plasma catecholamine levels and pharmacokinetics. *Acta Anaesthesiologica Scandinavica*, 25: 328-331.
40. Kates RE, Leier CV, (1978), Dobutamine pharmacokinetics in severe heart failure. *Clinical Pharmacology & Therapeutics*, 24: 537-541.
41. Abernethy DR, et al., (1981), Digoxin disposition in obesity: clinical pharmacokinetic investigation. *American Heart Journal*, 102: 740-744.
42. Sparr HJ, et al, (2007), Early Reversal of Profound Rocuronium-induced Neuromuscular Blockade by Sugammadex in a Randomized Multicenter Study: Efficacy, Safety, and Pharmacokinetics. *Anesthesiology*, 106: 935-943.